PTSD in Children and Adolescents

Review of Psychiatry Series
John M. Oldham, M.D.
Michelle B. Riba, M.D., M.S.
Series Editors

PTSD in Children and Adolescents

EDITED BY

Spencer Eth, M.D.

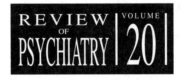

No. 1

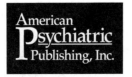

Washington, DC
London, England

Copyright © 2001 American Psychiatric Publishing, Inc.
04   03   02   01   4   3   2   1

ALL RIGHTS RESERVED
Manufactured in the United States of America on acid-free paper
First Edition

American Psychiatric Publishing, Inc.
1400 K Street, NW
Washington, DC 20005
www.appi.org

The correct citation for this book is

Eth S (editor): *PTSD in Children and Adolescents* (Review of Psychiatry Series, Volume 20, Number 1; Oldham JM and Riba MB, series editors). Washington, DC, American Psychiatric Publishing, 2001

Library of Congress Cataloging-in-Publication Data
PTSD in children and adolescents / edited by Spencer Eth.
    p. ; cm — (Review of Psychiatry ; v. 20, no. 1)
  Includes bibliographical references and index.
  ISBN 1-58562-026-2 (alk. paper)
    1. Post-traumatic stress disorder in children. 2. Teenagers—Mental health.
  [DNLM: 1. Stress Disorders, Post-Traumatic—diagnosis—Adolescence.
  2. Stress Disorders, Post-Traumatic—diagnosis—Child. 3. Stress
  Disorders, Post-Traumatic—therapy—Adolescence. 4. Stress Disorders,
  Post-Traumatic—therapy—Child. 5. Forensic Psychiatry—methods. 6.
  Psychotherapy—methods—Adolescence. 7. Psychotherapy—methods—
  Child.   WM 170 P975 2001] I. Title: Post-traumatic stress disorder in
  children and adolescents. II. Eth, Spencer, 1950- III. Review of psychiatry
  series ; v. 20, 1
    RJ506.P55 .P875 2001
    616.85'21—dc21

                            00-067404

British Library Cataloguing in Publication Data
A CIP record is available from the British Library.

*To my wife, Cheryl, a woman
of kindness and valor.*

Contents

Contributors   xi

Introduction to the Review of Psychiatry Series   xiii
John M. Oldham, M.D., and
Michelle B. Riba, M.D., M.S., Series Editors

Introduction: Childhood Trauma in Perspective   xvii
Spencer Eth, M.D.

Chapter 1

**Evaluation and Assessment of PTSD in
Children and Adolescents**   1
Evan B. Drake, Ph.D.
Sherry F. Bush, Ph.D.
Wilfred G. van Gorp, Ph.D.
Introduction   1
Issues in the Assessment of
    Children and Adolescents   1
Clinical Guidelines for Assessment   4
Recent Developments in Clinical Assessment   5
Multidimensional Approach to Assessment   15
Conclusions   26
References   27

Chapter 2

**Forensic Aspects of PTSD in
Children and Adolescents**   33
James E. Rosenberg, M.D.
Introduction   33
Diagnosis   34
Epidemiology   38
Genetics   39
Risk Factors in Various Settings   39

Psychophysiology   44
Assessment   45
PTSD and Memory   47
Treatment   50
Conclusions and Recommendations   51
References   54

Chapter 3

PTSD in Children and Adolescents in the
Juvenile Justice System   **59**

William Arroyo, M.D.

Introduction   59
Demographics   60
Mental Disorders   61
Posttraumatic Stress Disorder   62
Incarcerated Youth   63
Female Population   65
Predisposing Factors   65
Interventions   70
Special National Challenge   77
Summary   78
References   79

Chapter 4

Biological Treatment of PTSD in
Children and Adolescents   **87**

Soraya Seedat, M.B.
Dan J. Stein, M.B.

Diagnosis and Phenomenology   88
Neurobiologic Systems in PTSD   90
Biologic Treatments in Children and Adolescents   94
Assessing Outcome in Children and Adolescents   104
Quality of Life   105
Conclusions   105
References   107

Chapter 5

**Relationship Between Childhood Traumatic
Experiences and PTSD in Adults** 117

Rachel Yehuda, Ph.D.
Ilyse L. Spertus, Ph.D.
Julia A. Golier, M.D.

Introduction   117
Long-Term Consequences of Childhood
    Maltreatment—Sexual Abuse, Physical
    Abuse, Emotional Abuse, and/or Neglect   118
Challenges in Formulating a
    Model of the Effects of Early
    Child Maltreatment on the Adult   124
Long-Term Consequences of Single-Episode
    Traumatic Events: Preliminary Evidence   125
Prevalence of PTSD in Children and
    Adults Following Childhood Trauma   127
Impact of Early Maltreatment on
    Reaction to Subsequent Trauma and
    Risk of Revictimization   129
Biological Models of the Effects of Stress:
    The Centrality of Sensitization as a
    Mechanism of Permanent Stress Responses   132
Developmental Influences of
    Early Stress in Animals   133
Biological Consequences in Adults
    Who Experienced Trauma in Childhood   135
PTSD and Other Psychological
    Symptoms in Adults Who
    Survived the Holocaust as Children   141
Methodologic Considerations in the Study of
    the Long-Term Impact of Childhood Trauma   143
Summary and Conclusions   146
References   146

Index   **159**

Contributors

William Arroyo, M.D.
Clinical Assistant Professor, Psychiatry and Behavioral Sciences, Keck School of Medicine, University of Southern California, Los Angeles, California

Sherry F. Bush, Ph.D.
Assistant Professor, Department of Psychology, Fordham University, New York, New York

Evan B. Drake, Ph.D.
Chief, Neuropsychology Section, Department of Psychology, Mount Carmel Guild Behavioral Healthcare System, Catholic Community Services, Newark, New Jersey

Spencer Eth, M.D.
Professor and Vice Chairman, Department of Psychiatry and Behavioral Sciences, New York Medical College; and Medical Director, Behavioral Health Services, Saint Vincent Catholic Medical Centers, New York, New York

Julia A. Golier, M.D.
Traumatic Stress Studies Program, Department of Psychiatry, Mount Sinai School of Medicine, New York, New York

John M. Oldham, M.D.
Dollard Professor and Acting Chairman, Department of Psychiatry, Columbia University College of Physicians and Surgeons, New York, New York

Michelle B. Riba, M.D., M.S.
Associate Chair for Education and Academic Affairs, Department of Psychiatry, University of Michigan Medical School, Ann Arbor, Michigan

James E. Rosenberg, M.D.
Assistant Clinical Professor of Psychiatry, University of California–Los Angeles School of Medicine, Los Angeles, California; Director, Forensic Neuropsychiatry Medical Group, Inc., Westlake Village, California

Soraya Seedat, M.B.
Medical Research Council Unit on Anxiety Disorders, University of Stellenbosch, Cape Town, South Africa

Ilyse L. Spertus, Ph.D.
Traumatic Stress Studies Program, Department of Psychiatry, Mount Sinai School of Medicine, New York, New York

Dan J. Stein, M.B.
Medical Research Council Unit on Anxiety Disorders, University of Stellenbosch, Cape Town, South Africa, and University of Florida, Gainesville, Florida

Wilfred G. van Gorp, Ph.D.
Professor, Department of Psychiatry, Weill Medical College of Cornell University, New York, New York

Rachel Yehuda, Ph.D.
Traumatic Stress Studies Program, Department of Psychiatry, Mount Sinai School of Medicine, New York, New York

Introduction to the Review of Psychiatry Series

John M. Oldham, M.D., and
Michelle B. Riba, M.D., M.S., Series Editors

2001 REVIEW OF PSYCHIATRY SERIES TITLES

- *PTSD in Children and Adolescents*
  EDITED BY SPENCER ETH, M.D.
- *Integrated Treatment of Psychiatric Disorders*
  EDITED BY JERALD KAY, M.D.
- *Somatoform and Factitious Disorders*
  EDITED BY KATHARINE A. PHILLIPS, M.D.
- *Treatment of Recurrent Depression*
  EDITED BY JOHN F. GREDEN, M.D.
- *Advances in Brain Imaging*
  EDITED BY JOHN M. MORIHISA, M.D.

In today's rapidly changing world, the dissemination of information is one of its rapidly changing elements. Information virtually assaults us, and proclaimed experts abound. Witness, for example, the 2000 presidential election in the United States, during which instant opinions were plentiful about the previously obscure science of voting machines, the electoral college, and the meaning of the words of the highest court in the land. For medicine the situation is the same: the World Wide Web virtually bulges with health advice, treatment recommendations, and strident warnings about the dangers of this approach or that. Authoritative and reliable guides to help the consumer differentiate between sound advice and unsubstantiated opinion are hard to come by, and our patients and their families may be misled by bad information without even knowing it.

At no time has it been more important, then, for psychiatrists and other clinicians to be well informed, armed with the very latest findings, and well versed in evidence-based medicine. We have designed Volume 20 of the Review of Psychiatry Series with these trends in mind—to be, if you will, a how-to manual: how to accurately identify illnesses, how to understand where they come from and what is going wrong in specific conditions, how to measure the extent of the problem, and how to design the best treatment, especially for the particularly difficult-to-treat disorders.

The central importance of stress as a pathogen in major mental illness throughout the life cycle is increasingly clear. One form of stress is *trauma*. Extreme trauma can lead to illness at any age, but its potential to set the stage badly for life when severe trauma occurs during early childhood is increasingly recognized. In *PTSD in Children and Adolescents*, Spencer Eth and colleagues review the evidence from animal and human studies of the aberrations, both psychological and biological, that can persist throughout adulthood as a result of trauma experienced during childhood. Newer technologies have led to new knowledge of the profound nature of some of these changes, from persistently altered stress hormones to gene expression and altered protein formation. In turn, hypersensitivities result from this early stress-induced biological programming, so that cognitive and emotional symptom patterns emerge rapidly in reaction to specific environmental stimuli.

Nowhere in the field of medicine is technology advancing more rapidly than in brain imaging, generating a level of excitement that surely surpasses the historical moment when the discovery of the X ray first allowed us to noninvasively see into the living human body. The new imaging methods, fortunately, do not involve the risk of radiation exposure, and the capacity of the newest imaging machines to reveal brain structure and function in great detail is remarkable. Yet in many ways these techniques still elude clinical application, since they are expensive and increasingly complex to administer and interpret. John Morihisa has gathered a group of our best experts to discuss the latest developments in *Advances in Brain Imaging*, and the shift toward greater clinical utility is clear in their descriptions of these methods. Perhaps most intriguing is the promise that through these methods we can identify, before the onset of symptoms, those most at risk of developing psychiatric disorders, as discussed by Daniel Pine regarding childhood disorders and by Harold Sackeim regarding late-life depression.

Certain conditions, such as the somatoform and factitious disorders, can baffle even our most experienced clinicians. As Katharine Phillips points out in her foreword to *Somatoform and Factitious Disorders*, these disorders frequently go unrecognized or are misdiagnosed, and patients with these conditions may be seen more often in the offices of nonpsychiatric physicians than in those of psychiatrists. Although these conditions have been reported throughout the recorded history of medicine, patients with these disorders either are fully convinced that their problems are "physical" instead of "mental" or choose to present their problems that way. In this book, experienced clinicians provide guidelines to help identify the presence of the somatoform and factitious disorders, as well as recommendations about their treatment.

Treatment of all psychiatric disorders is always evolving, based on new findings and clinical experience; at times, the field has become polarized, with advocates of one approach vying with advocates of another (e.g., psychotherapy versus pharmacotherapy). Patients, however, have the right to receive the best treatment available, and most of the time the best treatment includes psychotherapy *and* pharmacotherapy, as detailed in *Integrated Treatment of Psychiatric Disorders*. Jerald Kay and colleagues propose the term *integrated treatment* for this approach, a recommended fundamental of treatment planning. Psychotherapy alone, of course, may be the best treatment for some patients, just as pharmacotherapy may be the mainstay of treatment for others, but in all cases there should be thoughtful consideration of a combination of these approaches.

Finally, despite tremendous progress in the treatment of most psychiatric disorders, there are some conditions that are stubbornly persistent in spite of the best efforts of our experts. John Greden takes up one such area in *Treatment of Recurrent Depres-*

sion, referring to recurrent depression as one of the most disabling disorders of all, so that, in his opinion, "a call to arms" is needed. Experienced clinicians and researchers review optimal treatment approaches for this clinical population. As well, new strategies, such as vagus nerve stimulation and minimally invasive brain stimulation, are reviewed, indicating the need to go beyond our currently available treatments for these seriously ill patients.

All in all, we believe that Volume 20 admirably succeeds in advising us how to do the best job that can be done at this point to diagnose, understand, measure, and treat some of the most challenging conditions that prompt patients to seek psychiatric help.

Introduction

Childhood Trauma in Perspective

Spencer Eth, M.D.

In 1985, the American Psychiatric Press published *Post-Traumatic Stress Disorder in Children* (Eth and Pynoos 1985b). This slim volume, which was edited by myself and Dr. Robert S. Pynoos, contained nine chapters, many of which were originally presented in a symposium during the May 1984 annual meeting of the American Psychiatric Association in Los Angeles, California. A success, the book rode a wave of interest in what was then a new concern for psychiatrists—the psychologic impact of traumatic events in the lives of children.

The monograph you are reading now, *PTSD in Children and Adolescents*, which is part of the 2001 *Review of Psychiatry* series, reflects the maturation of the field of "developmental psychotraumatology." Clinical practices in childhood trauma are today based on a wealth of research and case studies found in hundreds, if not thousands, of publications in the scientific literature. It is with a sense of pride for this progress that we contrast the respective states of knowledge captured in these two works.

Prior to the 1980 publication of the DSM-III (American Psychiatric Association 1980), posttraumatic stress disorder (PTSD) did not exist. Except, of course, that it did. For, unlike acquired immune deficiency syndrome (AIDS), PTSD is an affliction that has plagued mankind since our prehistoric ancestors were attacked by predatory animals, were devastated by natural disasters, and engaged in tribal warfare. Many authors have delighted in finding literary descriptions characteristic of PTSD in various fiction and nonfiction works dating back to Homer (Daly 1983).

The modern era of traumatic studies may be said to have begun with World War I, when soldiers were routinely exposed to death and devastation on an unprecedented scale. The term *shell shock* was applied to those soldiers who responded to combat with severe psychiatric symptoms. Although first believed to be an emotional manifestation of brain injury, shell shock came to be accepted as having a psychological etiology (Hynes 1997). Freud, having observed victims of shell shock, suggested that an unbearable situation could itself be pathologic. Contrary to his usual emphasis on regression to forbidden infantile fantasies, Freud reasoned that real-life trauma confronts the mind with affects too powerful to be assimilated, thereby overwhelming the stimulus barrier. In his final work, *Moses and Monotheism,* published at the time of his death in 1939, Freud conceptualized psychic trauma as composed of two types of symptoms: *positive effects,* which are fixations to the trauma and repetition compulsions, and *negative effects,* which are the defensive reactions of avoidance, inhibition, and phobia (Freud 1939/1962). These formulations are analogous to the DSM-III–defined symptom clusters of reexperiencing and numbing.

World War II, the European Holocaust, and the atomic bombing of Hiroshima highlighted the psychiatric sequela of massive psychic trauma. In particular, adult prisoners of war and survivors of the concentration camps were often found to be suffering from severe posttraumatic syndromes that persisted or worsened over the course of years despite intensive treatment (Krystal 1968). For the first time, there began to appear in the professional literature case reports of children who had been dislocated, orphaned, injured, or incarcerated during the war. Because of the broad range of age and circumstances of these children and the theoretical orientation and methodology of the authors, these papers failed to convey a consistent clinical picture. In retrospect, the data collected were probably overly dependent on information provided by parents and other secondary sources who may have wished to deny the gravity of the children's emotional pain. For example, Anna Freud failed to detect "signs of traumatic shock" in the youngsters in her war nursery (Freud and Burlingham 1943).

The first rigorous investigation of childhood trauma was conducted in the wake of the Vicksburg, Mississippi, tornado of December 1953. One week after the disaster, two child psychiatrists spoke with children, parents, and community members and then distributed questionnaires. They found a significant association between being severely disturbed and having been within the tornado's impact zone. They also noted the appearance of "tornado games" in some children's play (Bloch et al. 1956). In 1972 another child psychiatrist reported clinical observations of fears in 56 children whose Welsh school had been engulfed in an avalanche of slag (Lacey 1972).

A landmark series of studies arose from a West Virginia disaster—the February 1972 Buffalo Creek slag dam collapse and flood. The filing of a lawsuit by the downstream residents resulted in psychiatric evaluations of the plaintiffs, including 224 children. One early publication described the "after-trauma" vulnerabilities of those victims who were under 12 years of age at the time of the flood (Newman 1976). A 17-year follow-up of this group of children found PTSD in 7% (all female) compared with 32% who were retrospectively diagnosed as having PTSD in the aftermath of the flood (Green et al. 1994).

The last major pre-DSM-III child trauma study was Dr. Lenore Terr's work with the children of Chowchilla. In July 1976, 26 California schoolchildren and their bus driver were kidnapped and buried alive in a van for 16 hours before escaping. Dr. Terr initially interviewed the children and then later, in separate research projects, conducted follow-up interviews of the victims and a comparison with a matched group of children from a similar town as control subjects. These studies forcefully established that traumatized children exhibited a unique constellation of signs and symptoms that can be understood in the context of their struggles to master their experience (Terr 1979). One aspect of this data set became the basis of Terr's chapter in *Post-Traumatic Stress Disorder in Children* (Terr 1985). In another chapter, Benedek (1985) chronicled the professional hostility that greeted Dr. Terr's first presentation of her findings, a reaction reminiscent of the rejecting response to the early accounts of child abuse.

The introduction of the DSM-III in 1980 provided the name of a new disorder, *posttraumatic stress disorder*, and in so doing served to organize the field of traumatic stress. PTSD was defined by its diagnostic criteria, which consisted of a definition of the traumatic stressor and three clusters of symptoms: 1) reexperiencing of the trauma (such as intrusive memories and nightmares of the event); 2) numbing of responsiveness to or reduced involvement with the external world (such as detachment and constricted affect); and 3) arousal (such as exaggerated startle reactions and sleep disturbance).

The creation of the PTSD diagnosis has been viewed as politically driven by the vocal demands of two special interest factions and their supporters—American veterans of the Vietnam War and adult women rape victims (Leys 2000). The absence of children in these populations may perhaps explain why DSM-III was silent about how PTSD would appear in children. None of the new diagnostic criteria contained explicit references to children. Clinicians were left to wonder: Does PTSD exist during childhood as a specific disorder? If so, should it be assumed that the condition presents identically regardless of gender, age, and developmental phase?

Certain distinguished child mental health experts opined that this form of stress disorder is not markedly different from other emotional disorders not precipitated by severely traumatic experiences (Garmezy and Rutter 1985). A contrary position was asserted in *Post-Traumatic Stress Disorder in Children* (Eth and Pynoos 1985b), wherein the prevalence of PTSD in special populations of children was carefully demonstrated. Using the DSM-III adult criteria for PTSD, authors readily diagnosed the disorder in various groups of children at risk for exposure to traumatic events.

Arroyo and Eth (1985) interviewed child refugees from the civil wars that were endemic in Central America. Excellent studies of the phenomenology, prevalence, and course of PTSD in Southeast Asian child immigrants soon followed (Sack et al. 1999). The destructive legacy of the exposure to violence in children from war zones and certain inner-city neighborhoods is, by now, well established (Apfel and Simon 1996). In Chapter 3 of this book,

Dr. Arroyo extends this work by examining the role of trauma in the lives of juvenile offenders. Similarly, Nir (1985) described the presence of iatrogenic PTSD in young cancer patients, a line of inquiry that has been pursued further in the pediatric consultation-liaison field (Stuber et al. 1997).

Physical abuse and sexual abuse can be experienced as traumatic; however, these acts are often repeated many times over the course of years in a child's life. Green (1985) delineated the disturbed psychodynamics and family interactions in abusive homes, whereas Goodwin (1985) examined the occurrence of traumatic symptoms in incest victims. Since that time, Terr (1991) has proposed the existence of two types of childhood traumatic syndromes that reflect fundamental differences between children exposed to single traumatic events and those experiencing chronic, multiple traumas.

In 1987, DSM-III-Revised was published (American Psychiatric Association 1987). Unlike its predecessor, DSM-III, this new edition contained two "child-friendly" examples among the diagnostic criteria for PTSD. The reexperiencing symptom of recurrent and intrusive distressing recollections can be satisfied in young children through repetitive play, in which themes or aspects of the trauma are expressed, such as the "tornado games" mentioned earlier. The numbing of responsiveness criterion of markedly diminished interest in significant activities may be fulfilled in young children by the loss of recently acquired developmental skills such as toilet training.

DSM-IV (American Psychiatric Association 1994) is noteworthy for its revision of the stressor criterion from a traumatic event that is outside the range of usual human experience and would be markedly distressing to almost anyone to a traumatic event that involved actual or threatened death or a serious injury that involved intense fear, helplessness, or horror. This new criterion recognizes that in many locations around the world violence is endemic, such that traumatic events cannot be considered outside of the range of usual human experience. DSM-IV notes that in children, the experience of traumatic stress can be expressed by disorganized or agitated behavior. In addition, the reexperiencing symptom of distressing dreams of the traumatic event in children can take the form of frightening dreams without recognizable content (a night terror). DSM-IV also introduces *trauma-specific reenactment* as the child example of the reexperiencing symptom of acting or feeling as if the traumatic event were recurring.

DSM-III, DSM-III-R, and DSM-IV have no specific diagnostic category for traumatic grief, although the DSMs do contain a V-code for bereavement that can be used when the focus of clinical attention is a "normal" reaction to the death of a loved one. If the sadness associated with the death is more severe and persistent, a diagnosis of major depressive disorder may be made. Pynoos and Eth (1985) reviewed their work with children who witnessed acts of extreme violence involving a parent, including homicide and suicide. They further (Eth and Pynoos 1985a) described circumstances in which the grieving process of children was disrupted by the traumatic circumstances of a parent's death. An understanding of the interplay of trauma and grief is critical in order to help the affected child mourn successfully. Recently, Prigerson et al. (1999) devised and tested criteria for the condition of traumatic grief in adults, whereas Stoppelbein and Greening (2000) reported on symptoms of posttraumatic stress in parentally bereaved children and adolescents.

Frederick (1985) was a pioneer in the use of a standardized instrument (the reaction index) to measure the severity of traumatic symptoms in children. Rating scales have since proven invaluable in both their research applications and their clinical applications. In Chapter 1, Drake, Bush, and van Gorp present an overview of the evaluation of PTSD in children and adolescents that surveys various instruments shown to have value in assessing children and adolescents.

The language and metaphor of psychoanalysis informed much of the early literature on childhood trauma. Over the past decade, the construct chosen for understanding the traumatic process has been increasingly biologic (Pfefferbaum 1997). There is a sense that breakthroughs in delineating the neurophysiologic diathesis of trauma are already on the horizon (Heim et al. 2000). Although the targeted application of this progress to specific, biologically based therapies is premature, psychopharmacologic agents are in widespread use for treating traumatized children and adolescents both in the United States (American Academy of Child and Adolescent Psychiatry 1998) and abroad (Perrin et al. 2000). Seed-at and Stein provide a comprehensive review of the important role of medication in clinical practice in Chapter 4.

From the Buffalo Creek disaster (Lindy and Titchener 1983) to today's toxic torts (Harr 1995), litigation has been a catalyst in stimulating the study of traumatized children and adolescents. Furthermore, many clinicians have been called to testify as expert witnesses about PTSD. However, even psychiatrists well versed on the subject of trauma may feel uncomfortable with judicial procedures and intimidated in a courtroom setting. In Chapter 2, Rosenberg familiarizes the reader with issues that are especially pertinent to the practice of forensic psychiatry, such as the reliability of traumatic memories in children.

One question that is usually asked of the expert witness testifying about PTSD is the prognosis for the affected child or adolescent. Do we know enough about risk and resiliency factors to make informed predictions about the natural history of childhood PTSD? The life course of child survivors of the Holocaust (Kestenberg and Brenner 1996) has been extensively studied, but the generalizability of these findings is unclear. In Chapter 5, Yehuda, Spertus, and Golier offer a comprehensive analysis of the literature and their own work in addressing the relationship between early trauma exposure, biologic substrates, and the subsequent development of PTSD in adulthood.

It is indeed a blessing that the field of child and adolescent PTSD has been transformed from an uncharted territory to a community crowded with investigators, practitioners, and excitement (Sugar 1999; Yule 2000). This book should find its place as a roadmap for clinicians seeking to expand their horizons in treating traumatized youth.

References

American Academy of Child and Adolescent Psychiatry: Practice parameters for the assessment and treatment of children and adolescents with posttraumatic stress disorder. J Am Acad Child Adolesc Psychiatry 37(suppl):4S–26S, 1998

American Psychiatric Association: Diagnostic and Statistical Manual of Mental Disorders, 3rd Edition. Washington, DC, American Psychiatric Association, 1980

American Psychiatric Association: Diagnostic and Statistical Manual of Mental Disorders, 3rd Edition Revised. Washington, DC, American Psychiatric Association, 1987

American Psychiatric Association: Diagnostic and Statistical Manual of Mental Disorders, 4th Edition. Washington, DC, American Psychiatric Association, 1994

Apfel RJ, Simon B (eds): Minefields in their Hearts: the Mental Health of Children in War and Communal Violence. New Haven, CT, Yale University Press, 1996

Arroyo W, Eth S: Children traumatized by Central American warfare, in Post-Traumatic Stress Disorder in Children. Edited by Eth S, Pynoos RS. Washington, DC, American Psychiatric Press, 1985, pp 101–120

Benedek EP: Children and psychic trauma: a brief review of contemporary thinking, in Post-Traumatic Stress Disorder in Children. Edited by Eth S, Pynoos RS. Washington, DC, American Psychiatric Press, 1985, pp 1–16

Bloch DA, Silber E, Perry SE: Some factors in the emotional reactions of children to disaster. Am J Psychiatry 113:416–422, 1956

Daly RJ: Samuel Pepys and post-traumatic stress disorder. Br J Psychiatry 143:64–68, 1983

Eth S, Pynoos RS: Interaction of trauma and grief in childhood, in Post-Traumatic Stress Disorder in Children. Edited by Eth S, Pynoos RS. Washington, DC, American Psychiatric Association, 1985a, pp 169–186

Eth S, Pynoos RS (eds): Post-Traumatic Stress Disorder in Children. Washington, DC, American Psychiatric Press, 1985b

Frederick CJ: Children traumatized by catastrophic situations, in Post-Traumatic Stress Disorder in Children. Edited by Eth S, Pynoos RS. Washington, DC, American Psychiatric Association, 1985, pp 71–100

Freud A, Burlingham D: War and Children. London, England, Medical War Books, 1943

Freud S: Moses and Monotheism (1939), in The Standard Edition of the Complete Psychological Works of Sigmund Freud, Vol 20. Translated and edited by Strachey J. London, England, Hogarth Press, 1962

Garmezy N, Rutter M: Acute reactions to stress, in Child and Adolescent Psychiatry: Modern Approaches, 2nd Edition. Edited by Rutter M, Hersov L. Oxford, England, Blackwell Scientific, 1985, pp 152–176

Goodwin, J: Post-traumatic symptoms in incest victims, in Post-Traumatic Stress Disorder in Children. Edited by Eth S, Pynoos RS. Washington, DC, American Psychiatric Press, 1985, pp 155–168

Green AH: Children traumatized by physical abuse, in Post-Traumatic Stress Disorder in Children. Edited by Eth S, Pynoos RS. Washington, DC, American Psychiatric Press, 1985, pp 133–154

Green BL, Grace MC, Vary MG, et al: Children of disaster in the second decade: a 17-year follow-up of Buffalo Creek survivors. J Am Acad Child Adolesc Psychiatry 33:71–79, 1994

Harr J: A Civil Action. New York, Random House, 1995

Heim C, Newport DJ, Heit S, et al: Pituitary–adrenal and autonomic responses to stress in women after sexual and physical abuse in childhood. JAMA 284:592–597, 2000

Hynes S: The Soldiers' Tale: Bearing Witness to Modern War. New York, Penguin, 1997

Kestenberg JS, Brenner I: The Last Witness: The Child Survivor of the Holocaust. Washington, DC, American Psychiatric Press, 1996

Krystal H (ed): Massive Psychic Trauma. New York, International Universities Press, 1968

Lacey GN: Observations on Aberfan. J Psychosom Res 16:257–260, 1972

Leys R: Trauma: A Genealogy. Chicago, IL, University of Chicago Press, 2000

Lindy JD, Titchener J: "Acts of God and man": long-term character change in survivors of disasters and the law. Behavioral Sciences and the Law 1:85–96, 1983

Newman CJ: Children of disaster: clinical observations at Buffalo Creek. Am J Psychiatry 133:306–312, 1976

Nir Y: Post-traumatic stress disorder in children with cancer, in Post-Traumatic Stress Disorder in Children. Edited by Eth S, Pynoos RS. Washington, DC, American Psychiatric Press, 1985, pp 121–132

Perrin S, Smith P, Yule W: Practitioner review: the assessment and treatment of post-traumatic stress disorder in children and adolescents. J Child Psychol Psychiatry 41:277–289, 2000

Pfefferbaum B: Posttraumatic stress disorder in children: a review of the past 10 years. J Am Acad Child Adolesc Psychiatry 36:1503–1511, 1997

Prigerson HG, Shear MK, Jacobs SC, et al: Consensus criteria for traumatic grief: a preliminary empirical test. Br J Psychiatry 44:67–73, 1999

Pynoos RS, Eth S: Children traumatized by witnessing acts of personal violence: homicide, rape, or suicide behavior, in Post-Traumatic Stress Disorder in Children. Edited by Eth S, Pynoos RS. Washington, DC, American Psychiatric Press, 1985, pp 17–44

Sack WH, Him C, Dickason D: Twelve-year follow-up study of Khmer youths who suffered massive war trauma as children. J Am Acad Child Adolesc Psychiatry 38:1173–1179, 1999

Stoppelbein L, Greening L: Posttraumatic stress symptoms in parentally bereaved children and adolescents. J Am Acad Child Adolesc Psychiatry 39:1112–1119, 2000

Stuber ML, Kazak AK, Meeske K, et al: Predictions of posttraumatic stress symptoms in childhood cancer survivors. Pediatrics 100:958–964, 1997

Sugar M (ed): Trauma and Adolescence. Madison, CT, International Universities Press, 1999

Terr LC: Children of Chowchilla: a study of psychic trauma. Psychoanalytic Study of the Child 34:552–623, 1979

Terr LC: Children traumatized in small groups, in Post-Traumatic Stress Disorder in Children. Edited by Eth S, Pynoos RS. Washington, DC, American Psychiatric Press, 1985, pp 45–70

Terr LC: Childhood traumas: an outline and overview. Am J Psychiatry 148:10–20, 1991

Yule W: Children and Traumatic Stress. New York, John Wiley and Sons, 2000

Chapter 1

Evaluation and Assessment of PTSD in Children and Adolescents

Evan B. Drake, Ph.D.
Sherry F. Bush, Ph.D.
Wilfred G. van Gorp, Ph.D.

Introduction

Posttraumatic stress disorder (PTSD) as a psychiatric diagnosis was formally introduced in DSM-III in 1980 by the American Psychiatric Association. In the past two decades, there has been increased awareness of the prevalence and clinical manifestations of the disorder in children and adolescents. The aim of this chapter is to provide the reader with a greater understanding of the clinical issues in, and an approach to, the evaluation of a child or adolescent at risk for PTSD. To this end, we review recently developed assessment methods of PTSD in children and adolescents and present an evaluation strategy and assessment method that comprises a comprehensive approach to the assessment of symptoms most prevalent in PTSD as well as those most appropriate in making a clinical diagnosis of the disorder.

Issues in the Assessment of Children and Adolescents

Diagnostic Criteria and Associated Symptoms

In DSM-IV (American Psychiatric Association 1994), the essential feature of PTSD is the development of a set of characteristic symptoms and responses after exposure to an extreme traumatic stressor or event. This characteristic cluster of symptoms can be summarized as follows: persistent reexperiencing of the event or stressor; persistent avoidance of triggers or reminders of the event; numbing of general responsiveness; and persistent symptoms of arousal (Pfefferbaum 1997). The DSM-IV diagnostic criteria include specific modifiers for children regarding their response and symptoms. Recurrent or intrusive thoughts about the experience may be expressed in repetitive play, as a form of rumination. Whereas having recurrent distressing dreams of the event is one of the diagnostic criteria for adults, children can experience frightening dreams that are without recognizable content. Symptoms more commonly seen in adults, such as dissociative flashbacks and reliving of the experience, may be expressed through trauma-specific reenactment in children.

Developmental Issues

The evaluation and assessment of children and adolescents for features of PTSD present a constellation of complex and unique challenges, due in part to the ongoing development of the child. Therefore, it is critical to evaluate the child or adolescent with his or her developmental context in mind; this is especially true when evaluating young children because the chronic course of PTSD can disrupt emotional development (Nader and Pynoos 1993; Perrin et al. 2000; Pfefferbaum 1997; Terr 1991). In addition, the nature of the stress-inducing event and the child's subjective experience of the trauma are influential factors in the expression of PTSD symptoms and are to some degree developmentally dependent. Time factors, such as time since the trauma occurred, are also relevant in the evaluation process. Effects of the traumatic experience, particularly if recent, can limit the evaluation process itself because of resistant and/or defensive behaviors. Developmental and psychosocial factors such as age, cognitive functioning, capacity for identifying or labeling emotions, verbal expressive ability, cultural background, gender, social competence, and familial support can further influence diagnosis and the manifestation of the disorder.

The research literature on childhood PTSD is diverse in terms of precipitating events studied (e.g., war, floods, school violence, bombings, physical abuse, sexual abuse). In contrast, the literature focusing on the clinical assessment of PTSD in children and adolescents is rather limited. There are relatively few validated, published, and accessible measures specifically designed to diagnose PTSD in children and adolescents based specifically on DSM-IV criteria. As a result, many researchers and clinicians have used instruments developed to assess broader areas of functioning and/or psychologic dysfunction, such as social adjustment, behavioral disorders, anxiety, memory, attention deficits, and depression, and have adapted adult measures of PTSD for use with children

Comorbidity and Age-Specific Symptoms in Assessment

Age-specific symptoms of regressed behavior, repetitive play, school refusal, loss of acquired developmental abilities, anxiety in strange situations, and diminished future expectations are common in children and adolescents with PTSD (C.J. Newman 1976; Pynoos and Eth 1985; Terr 1994). In young children, fears of the dark, nightmares, and interrupted sleep cycle may be prevalent (Terr 1994) and anxiety and fear may be exhibited that are not directly related to the trauma or event. Irritability, social avoidance, separation anxiety, diminished attention, and memory problems have been observed in children and adolescents. Not surprisingly, the rates of psychiatric comorbidity with PTSD are high and anxiety and depression are common. Likewise, cognitive problems that compromise attention, memory, and academic performance have also been identified. Adolescents who are victims of physical and sexual abuse may be at even greater risk for behavioral and social difficulties than for PTSD (Pelcovitz et al. 1994). Reviews of the accompanying cognitive, emotional, and behavioral disorders in children at risk for PTSD are presented by Pelcovitz and Kaplan (1996), Perrin et al. (2000), and Pfefferbaum (1997).

Clinical and Forensic Issues

Because PTSD must follow an extreme stressor or traumatic event to be diagnosed according to DSM-IV criteria, an evaluation is often requested after such events. However, relying exclusively on DSM-IV symptom characteristics to mandate and guide the evaluation can restrict the diagnosis of comorbid conditions, preexisting psychologic variables, and underlying psychopathology. Furthermore, relying only on DSM-IV criteria can result in an evaluation in which a tail of symptoms wags a diagnostic dog, thus finding only that for which one is looking. Therefore, it is of paramount importance that the clinician take a broad view of diagnostic possibilities, particularly in the absence of a clearly defined stressor.

Of particular importance in forensic settings is the issue of symptom validity and motivation. Although most research literature has focused on settings in which the causal event is not in question, this is not necessarily the case in forensic, legal, or criminal settings. Thus, it is of the utmost importance that measures of symptom validity and motivation be administered. Because most PTSD measures were developed in the context of research, very few contain such scales. The one known exception is the Trauma Symptom Checklist for Children (Briere 1996a). If the veracity of the symptoms reported comes into question, a measure that assesses validity must be included even if not specific to PTSD, such as the Minnesota Multiphasic Personality Inventory-Adolescent (MMPI-A; Butcher et al. 1992) or the Personality Inventory for Children (PIC; Wirt et al. 1990).

Clinical Guidelines for Assessment

In 1998, the American Academy of Child and Adolescent Psychiatry (AACAP) published "Practice Parameters for the Assessment and Treatment of Children and Adolescents with Posttraumatic Stress Disorder" (Cohen et al. 1998), which made three major recommendations for the assessment of PTSD in children and adolescents: 1) the use of clinical interviewing with specific focus on PTSD symptoms; 2) recognition of developmental influences; and 3) implementation of trauma-focused treatment interventions. These practice parameters provide a basic framework for the evaluation of children and adolescents at risk for PTSD. In addition to the minimum requirements set forth by the AACAP, we recommend and outline below a comprehensive, multifactorial, and multidisciplinary approach that takes into consideration the myriad known—as well as potential—variables that may compromise a young person's immediate and future well-being. An essential element of this model is the use of reliable and valid assessment tools.

Recent Developments in Clinical Assessment

Increased interest in the area of PTSD in children and adolescents has resulted in an explosion of instruments for both clinical and research use. However, as noted by other authors (Ruggiero and McLeer 2000; Saigh et al. 2000), a continuing issue plaguing the field is the paucity of well-validated, standardized, and readily available assessment instruments. Perhaps in response to these needs, new instruments have been developed in recent years and older measures have been revised to include information on reliability and validity. This chapter does not attempt to review all extant PTSD measures. Rather, recently developed and promising measures with available psychometric data are reviewed. For measures and articles published through 1996, we refer the reader to other excellent sources such as Carlson (1997), Nader (1997), and McNally (1991).

Child and Adolescent Psychiatric Assessment: Life Events Section and PTSD Module (CAPA-PTSD)

The Child and Adolescent Psychiatric Assessment: Life Events Section and PTSD Module (CAPA-PTSD; Costello et al. 1998) is a recently developed, comprehensive, structured child and/or parent clinical interview for use in both epidemiologic and clinical settings. The CAPA-PTSD was developed as an interviewer-based measure that would detail the timing of events and the onset of symptoms to better assess causality and the relationship among other stress-related disorders; measure additional non–Criterion A (actual or threatened death or serious injury to physical integrity of self or others) stressors that might contribute to psychiatric vulnerability and comorbidity; assess PTSD symptoms in excess of DSM-IV criteria that might be of clinical and research interest; and be suitable for both clinical and research settings (Costello et al. 1998). Because the CAPA-PTSD was validated in children ages 9–17, the authors caution against its use for children younger than 8. The time necessary to administer the Life Events Section and the PTSD module can range from 10 minutes for a nontraumatized child to 1 hour for a child who has experienced multiple traumas and is currently symptomatic.

The PTSD modules were designed to be used in conjunction with the Life Events Section (LES) of the CAPA (Angold et al. 1995). Rather than functioning solely as a screening device, the LES probes for two sets of stressors: 1) extreme stressors or "high-magnitude events," such as witnessing a traumatic event or being in a serious accident, as are necessary for the diagnosis of PTSD and 2) "low-magnitude events," such as parental divorce, that might increase psychiatric vulnerability in children but do not meet diagnostic criteria for PTSD. The LES contains protocols to minimize the number of full interviews administered that do not lead to diagnosis, thus saving clinicians' time and, more important, reducing the chances of false-positive diagnoses. The LES accomplishes this by first restricting low-magnitude events that qualify for evaluation to those occurring 3 months before the interview and second by including screening questions that establish whether the child has the three core symptoms of PTSD: reexperiencing/painful recall, hypervigilance, and avoidance. If the core symptoms are present and if the child or parent specifically links them to the trauma, then the full PTSD module is administered. Low-magnitude stressors are included on the theoretical grounds that events that trigger PTSD in children may not be identical to those that trigger the disorder in adults.

The full administration of the PTSD modules involves several steps. First, inquiries are made about multiple acute emotional and somatic responses to the event. Second, the precise nature of

Criterion B (reexperiencing), C (avoidance/numbing), and D (hyperarousal) symptoms are explored, including date of onset for Criterion E (duration). CAPA-PTSD requires distress for Criterion B–D symptoms to be coded, so a separate rating for Criterion F (clinically significant distress or impairment in social/occupational/other functioning) is not necessary. Third, the interviewer asks about other, extra–DSM-IV behavior such as survivor guilt. The interviewer also inquires about the patient's functioning with parents, siblings, peers, and important others. Scoring of the CAPA-PTSD is currently an impediment for use of the scale by clinicians because the interview results must be entered into a computer scoring program for diagnoses to be generated.

In the initial validation study of 58 parent–child pairs, the reliability of the screening items was fair for children ($\kappa=0.45$–0.51) and fair to excellent for parents ($\kappa=0.40$–0.79). Detailed interviews were conducted with a total of nine families, and intraclass correlations for the total symptoms scale were 0.94 for children and 0.99 for parents. The standardization and reliability data for the full PTSD module is promising, as are the theoretical bases of the measure. If the computer scoring program is made available to clinicians, then the CAPA-PTSD may well prove to be a useful tool in the clinical assessment of PTSD.

Clinician-Administered PTSD Scale for Children and Adolescents for DSM-IV (CAPS-CA)

The Clinician-Administered PTSD Scale for Children and Adolescents for DSM-IV (CAPS-CA; Nader et al. 1998) is a detailed, structured clinical interview developed by the National Center for PTSD and the University of California–Los Angeles (UCLA) Trauma Psychiatry Program and distributed by the Hitchcock Foundation of Dartmouth-Hitchcock Medical Center. Originally developed for use with DSM-III/DSM-III-R (American Psychiatric Association 1987) criteria, the CAPS-CA was revised for DSM-IV criteria in October 1998. The CAPS-CA rates both the frequency and the intensity of PTSD symptoms and provides rating sheets with pictorial scales to help depict more abstract concepts, including frequency (calendars marked with Xs), intensity-problems (cartoon figures with facial and somatic expressions), and intensity-feelings (facial expressions). The CAPS-CA also assesses the frequency and intensity of PTSD-associated symptoms that are not part of the DSM-IV diagnostic criteria.

Before administering the full CAPS-CA, the clinician completes the Life Events Checklist (LEC), an inventory of traumatic events, to determine the presence and number of traumas the child has experienced. Up to three traumatic events can be investigated and recorded using the LEC and CAPS-CA. After the presence of a traumatic event has been established, the clinician can interview the child about the event, particularly regarding issues of fear and terror, helplessness, horror, and agitation, to determine if Criterion A is met. The screening of events for Criterion A is necessary to exclude upsetting but not life-threatening or body-integrity–threatening events. Although there is some controversy as to what constitutes a PTSD-precipitating trauma in childhood, such as parental divorce, frequent moves, and bullying, we concur with Nader (1997) that, although there apparently may be similar symptom constellations between children exposed to clear life- or integrity-threatening trauma and children exposed to divorce, there are qualitative differences in the symptoms with which these children present. Thus, although children may exhibit PTSD-like symptoms of anxiety and depression secondary to understandably upsetting events, their symptoms do not meet current diagnostic criteria for PTSD and their difficulties might be better described by other diagnostic categories.

If the trauma(s) meets Criterion A, the clinician proceeds with the diagnostic section of the evaluation. The first 17 items of the CAPS-CA systematically assess for all Criterion B, C, and D symptoms. The duration of current symptoms is then established, followed by items assessing Criterion F. After Criterion F has been probed, the clinician is asked to provide global ratings for the validity of responses, severity of symptoms, and overall improvement. Although the clinician is asked to rate response validity, this is wholly dependent on clinical judgment rather than empirically established standards or base rates of item endorsement. Thus, it represents a clinical impression rather than empirical evidence of validity. The CAPS-CA concludes with three meta-questions aimed at helping children begin to reframe the traumas and focus on adaptation: How the trauma has affected their lives, what has helped them feel better, and what do they do to feel better when they are feeling bad?

The National Center for PTSD continues to gather data on the psychometric properties of the CAPS-CA but has not yet published its findings. However, in a recent study, Newman et al. (1998/2000) administered the CAPS-CA to 50 incarcerated adolescent males and found internal consistency α coefficients of 0.81, 0.75, and 0.79 for the Criterion B, C, and D symptom clusters, respectively. Although reliability and validity data remain sparse, the CAPS-CA provides a detailed, easily administered structured interview that will guide the clinician through all aspects of assessing PTSD and assist in the diagnosis of the disorder.

Children's PTSD Inventory (CPTSDI)

The Children's PTSD Inventory (CPTSDI; Saigh et al. 2000) is a rapidly administered interview developed to assess for PTSD in children and adolescents ages 7–18. This measure appears to have undergone extensive test development that included having experimental items paraphrased by children for increased clarity; field-testing; review by three psychologists who served on the DSM-IV PTSD advisory group; and review by a panel that included a minority and a nonminority school psychologist, two child psychiatrists, two elementary school teachers, and a minority social worker. The feedback from these sources was incorporated through the addition, modification, and deletion of items. The resulting iteration of the CPTSDI contains five subtests consistent with current diagnostic criteria: exposure, reexperiencing, avoidance, hyperarousal, and degree of distress.

The inventory begins with a preface that includes examples of traumatic incidents. All instructions for administration and scoring are incorporated into the inventory form. The first subtest of the CPTSDI contains four questions about potential exposure to trauma and four questions about reactivity during the trauma. If the child or adolescent fails to meet criteria for trauma exposure or reactivity, the interview is terminated. If the criteria are met, the interview continues through the subtests for reexperiencing

(11 items), avoidance and numbing (16 items), hyperarousal (7 items), and significant distress (5 items) as well as items to determine the duration of distress for endorsed symptoms. Each item of the inventory is scored dichotomously for the presence or absence of the symptom and, in turn, each subtest is scored dichotomously for meeting or not meeting DSM-IV symptom cluster criteria (e.g., one or more of the reexperiencing symptoms [Criterion B] must be present for the reexperiencing subtest to be scored positively). The CPTSDI yields five possible diagnoses: PTSD Negative, Acute PTSD, Chronic PTSD, Delayed Onset PTSD, and No Diagnosis. Bachelor's level individuals can administer the CPTSDI after 2 hours of professionally supervised analog training and feedback, and administration requires between 5 and 20 minutes depending on the trauma history of the child.

A validation study for the CPTSDI was conducted with 82 stress-exposed and 22 nonexposed youths recruited from an urban psychiatric and medical center (Saigh et al. 2000). Internal consistency across the subtests ranged from Cronbach's α of 0.53 to 0.89, with α scores below 0.80 occurring only in the four-item Situational Reactivity subtest ($\alpha=0.53$) and the five-item Significant Impairment subtest ($\alpha=0.69$). The internal consistency of the entire 43-item scale (diagnosis level) was extremely high (Cronbach's $\alpha=0.95$). Interrater reliability, as measured by intraclass correlations, was 0.88 or better for all subtests and 0.98 at the diagnostic level; as measured by Cohen's κ, it ranged from 0.66 to 1.00 level for subtests, with κ scores below 0.90 occurring only in Situational Reactivity ($\kappa=0.66$) and Reexperiencing ($\kappa=0.84$). Cohen's κ for the overall diagnosis was 0.96. There was diagnostic disagreement between the two independent administrations on only 2 of the 104 cases. These findings indicate that the CPTSDI provides a relatively rapid and reliable measure for diagnosing PTSD in children age 7 or older.

Child Posttraumatic Stress Reaction Index (CPTS-RI)

The Child Posttraumatic Stress Reaction Index (CPTS-RI; Frederick 1985; Frederick et al. 1992) is the most widely used instrument for assessing PTSD in children. This 20-item measure can be used both as a self-report instrument for older children and adolescents and as the basis for a semistructured interview in younger children or when more thorough inquiry is desired (Nader 1997). The index's items correspond to most Criterion B, C, and D symptoms and are rated on a 5-point scale ranging from 0 (none of the time) to 4 (most of the time). The possible range of resulting scores is 0–80, with scores less than 7 classified as no PTSD, scores of 7–9 classified as mild PTSD, scores of 10–12 classified as moderate PTSD, and scores greater than 12 classified as severe PTSD (Nader et al. 1990; Pynoos et al. 1987). Administration of the CPTS-RI takes between 20 and 45 minutes. The self-report format is suitable for children at least 8 years of age, and no minimum age is given for the semistructured format (Perrin et al. 2000). According to Nader (1997), two criticisms have been made about the CPTS-RI: 1) that it does not inquire about all DSM-IV symptoms and queries some symptoms more than once and 2) that items inquire about the enjoyment of activities, sleep, and concentration rather than about symptoms in these areas, which hinders diagnostic efficacy. Nader recommends that the clinician make additional note of the level of symptoms for each of these questions. Clinicians who choose to use the CPTS-RI should keep in mind that the symptom constellations are incomplete.

In several investigations, the CPTS-RI has been shown to be internally consistent and to relate closely to clinical judgments of PTSD severity (Frederick 1985; Nader et al. 1990; Pynoos et al. 1987). The original version of the CPTS-RI was standardized on 750 children and 1,350 adults exposed to stressful events (Frederick 1985) and the correlation between the CPTS-RI and diagnosed cases of PTSD was 0.91 for children and 0.95 for adults. A study of the factor structure of the CPTS-RI found three identifiable factors: 1) reexperiencing/numbing, 2) fear/anxiety, and 3) concentration/sleep, with Cronbach's αs of 0.80, 0.69, and 0.68, respectively (Pynoos et al. 1987). In a follow-up to the 1987 study, inter-item agreement was 94% with a Cohen's κ of 0.89 (Nader et al. 1990). However, studies that published reliability data on the CPTS-RI used the version developed for DSM-III-R criteria, not the more recently developed version for DSM-IV. This raises some concern about the psychometric properties of the newer revision. However, given that the symptoms clusters and descriptions have not changed from DSM-III-R to DSM-IV, it is reasonable to assume that the DSM-IV version has similar psychometric properties.

For the clinician, the CPTS-RI represents a well-established, highly utilized measure of PTSD that was specifically developed to assess the disorder in children. Thus, although it does have its noted limitations, the clinician using CPTS-RI for clinical evaluations would be in good company.

Schedule for Affective Disorders and Schizophrenia for School-Age Children— Present and Lifetime Version (K-SADS-PL)

The Kiddie Schedule for Affective Disorders and Schizophrenia for School-Age Children—Present and Lifetime Version (K-SADS-PL; Kaufman et al. 1997) is a revision and adaptation of the original K-SADS (Chambers et al. 1985) that includes a lifetime psychiatric history, previously omitted diagnostic categories including PTSD, and screening questions to allow interviewers to bypass nonsymptomatic areas. As reported in its validation study (Kaufman et al. 1997), the K-SADS-PL is highly dependent on the skill and training of the clinician for diagnostic accuracy and therefore requires intensive training in the use of the instrument, diagnostic classification, and differential diagnosis. Thus, although it is an excellent measure for use in childhood PTSD research, we do not recommend that clinicians who have not been specifically trained in its administration use it in clinical applications.

Darryl, A Cartoon-Based Measure of Cardinal Posttraumatic Stress Symptoms in School-Age Children

Darryl is a clinician-administered assessment device that uses cartoons to help children describe their experiences and that assesses all of the cardinal DSM-IV symptoms of PTSD. It was developed by Neugebauer et al. (1999) to be an independent measure of posttraumatic symptoms and as a possible screening instrument for children at risk for PTSD. Furthermore, given the urban child's potential for multiple exposures to traumatic events, Darryl was designed such that symptoms are not necessarily anchored to one traumatic event.

Darryl consists of 19 items measuring the three symptom clusters of PTSD. Seven of the items measure reexperiencing, seven measure avoidance/affective blunting, and five measure hyperarousal. Each item features Darryl, an 8- or 9-year-old boy of indeterminate ethnicity, in a cartoon depicting a PTSD symptom. The traumatic event or events are described as "something scary" that happened to the child, which was thought to be sufficiently open-ended language to allow the child to link symptoms to one or multiple events. For each cartoon, the clinician reads a script describing the symptom. The child then chooses one of three responses—"never," "some of the time," or "a lot of the time"—each of which has an accompanying graph of a thermometer to further the child's comprehension. According to the authors, the wording and cartoon depictions make Darryl suitable for children 6 years of age or older.

The initial reliability and validity of the Darryl instrument was assessed using 110 children born in 1985 and 1986 at a urban hospital located in a high crime and poverty area. The 110 children in the study were ages 7–9 years; 56% were boys; and 94% were African-American. In this sample, 93.6% of the children reported witnessing one or more violent events, and 26.9% reported being victims of violence. The overall internal consistency of Darryl, as measured by Cronbach's α, was 0.92 and was 0.78, 0.83, and 0.80, respectively, for the three subscales (reexperiencing, avoidance, and arousal). To assess construct validity, the clinicians correlated the children's scores on a traumatic event exposure scale with their Darryl scores. Among other findings, the sum of the event scores was significantly correlated with the summed symptom scores. Additionally, the proportion of children with "probable PTSD" (at least one reexperiencing symptom, more than two avoidance symptoms, and more than one arousal symptom) increased significantly with increasing exposure scores.

Future field-testing is planned for Darryl using a more heterogeneous population. In addition, an elaboration of Darryl, with additional probes for symptom duration and distress/social impairment, is planned so that it may be used directly as a diagnostic tool.

Trauma Symptom Checklist for Children (TSCC)

The self-report Trauma Symptom Checklist for Children (TSCC; Briere 1996a, 1996b) is one of the few, if not the only, commercially published trauma inventories. The standardization of the TSCC was based on a sample of 3,008 nonclinical children ages 7–17 from diverse racial, economic, and regional backgrounds. The size of the normative sample sets the TSCC apart substantially from almost all other PTSD measures as does the fact that it was standardized on ostensibly "normal" children. The TSCC is appropriate for use with children ages 8–16. It can be administered in either of two forms—the full 54-item TSCC, which includes 10 items for assessing sexual symptoms and preoccupations, or the 44-item TSCC-A, which makes no reference to sexual issues. Each item of the TSCC is scored along a 4-point scale, ranging from 0 (never) to 3 (lots of times). The TSCC yields two validity scales and five clinical scales, all of which have a mean T-score of 50 and a standard deviation of 1. As with the MMPI scales, a T-score of 65 is considered clinically elevated (with the exception of the Hyperresponse [HYP] validity scale and the Sexual Concerns [SC] clinical scale).

The TSCC validity scales consist of Underresponse (UND) and Hyperresponse (HYP). UND measures whether a child is passively resisting the test by indiscriminately marking "0s" and consists of the 10 TSCC items that least frequently received ratings of 0 in the normative sample. These items include behaviors, thoughts, or feelings that most children do not deny, such as daydreaming. The Hyperresponse scale (HYP) was developed to screen for random endorsement of high-frequency scores (those marked with a "3"). The HYP scale consists of the number of "3" ratings on the eight TSCC items that were the most infrequently endorsed by the normative sample. An elevated HYP scale indicates a generalized overendorsing style, a desire to appear very distressed or dysfunctional, or a "cry for help."

The six clinical scales of the TSCC consist of Anxiety (ANX), Depression (DEP), Anger (ANG), Posttraumatic Stress (PTS), Dissociation (DIS), and Sexual Concerns (SC). In general, these scales measure symptoms associated with their named domains. Additionally, the DIS and SC can be subdivided into subscales that were developed using both content analysis and principal components analysis. With the exception of SC ($\alpha=0.77$) and HYP ($\alpha=0.66$), the internal consistency αs of all scales range from 0.82 to 0.89. The clinical scales of the TSCC do not overlap directly with DSM-IV criteria. According to Briere (1996a, 1996b), the TSCC was developed as a self-report measure of posttraumatic distress and related symptoms, not as a stand-alone diagnostic tool. For example, the PTS scale contains more intrusive symptoms than avoidance or hyperarousal symptoms, and should not be considered a comprehensive measurement of PTSD. The manual of the TSCC reemphasizes that the diagnosis of PTSD can be made only in a face-to-face interview using the criteria of the DSM-IV. With those caveats in mind, the substantial normative base of the TSCC and its inclusion of validity scales should make it a welcome, if not necessary, addition to any clinical assessment of PTSD.

Although no instrument can take the place of the face-to-face psychiatric interview for the diagnosis of PTSD, the instruments reviewed above and interviews do provide a necessary and vital component for the comprehensive, multidimensional clinical assessment of PTSD in children and adolescents described below.

Multidimensional Approach to Assessment

As mentioned previously, the nature of PTSD demands a multidimensional approach in the evaluation process. This approach includes the assessment of current emotional functioning and symptoms, developmental history and status, and cognitive functioning to fully assess the constellation of physiologic, psychologic, and social symptoms and behaviors associated with the disorder, which has been described elsewhere as an "abnormal reaction to an abnormal event" (Perrin et al. 2000; Yehuda and McFarlane 1995). Therefore, evaluation of children and adolescents demands consideration of the dynamic interplay for these factors, which can only be adequately captured in a multidimensional evaluation.

A comprehensive clinical PTSD evaluation process involves a team of medical and mental health professionals who each contribute specialized expertise. A neuropsychologist, for example, can work with the psychiatrist in designing a comprehensive assessment battery and administering formal assessment measures to provide the objective data needed in diagnosis and, later, for treatment planning. The evaluation process may include assessment of cognitive, emotional/behavioral, personality, developmental, social-adaptive, and academic functioning. In the following section we outline the steps involved in this comprehensive assessment process.

Clinical Interviews/Behavioral Observations

Before the face-to-face interview with the child, the clinician's task begins with investigating the facts about the nature of the trauma, the timing of the event, initial reactions observed by parents, individuals involved, and any subsequent psychiatric interventions.

The AACAP practice parameters mentioned earlier specifically emphasize the importance of the clinical interview as the foundation of the clinical assessment (Cohen et al. 1998). Interviews with the child or adolescent and his or her parent(s) yield information about life before the event, recall of the traumatic event experienced or witnessed, immediate versus delayed reactions, and behavioral and emotional functioning subsequent to the event. Most important, the interview provides an opportunity for the child to describe and further process the traumatic event in his or her own terms. Like the evaluation itself, the purpose of the interview should not be solely to assess whether the child meets DSM-IV diagnostic criteria for PTSD but should focus on obtaining critical objective and subjective information about the child's overall functioning in addition to his or her symptoms. This approach provides the clinician with a contextual framework within which PTSD symptoms can be differentiated from developmental, cognitive, and social-adaptive factors and facilitates greater understanding and identification of disorders that often accompany PTSD. Specific aspects of interviewing children, adolescents, and parents are presented below.

Clinical Interview of Parents

The clinical interview of parents should focus on the child's overall functioning both before and after the trauma. In their review of the assessment and treatment of childhood PTSD, Perrin et al. (2000) provided guidelines for interviewing parents as part of a PTSD evaluation. For example, the clinician may find it helpful to meet with parents separately and not in the presence of their child. A full developmental and medical history should be obtained from the parents before the interview with the child because this information may influence the evaluation process. During the parent interview, the clinician should also gain an understanding of family structure, familial history of psychiatric disorders, the child's personality and social functioning before the trauma, and any history of separations, abuse, or familial conflict. The parents should also be questioned about the child's treatment after the trauma and his or her emotional functioning since the event. It is also important to gain a sense of the parents' account of the trauma and how the trauma has affected the familial structure. Finally, the clinician should be aware that parents often underestimate and underreport their child's distress after trauma (Earls et al. 1988; McFarlane 1987; Pynoos and Eth 1986). Clinician guidelines and model interviews appropriate for the assessment of PTSD are available in *Clinical and Forensic Interviewing of Children and Families* (Sattler 1997).

Several structured parent interviews have been developed to help the clinician assess parents' impressions of their child's emotional functioning, and a small sample of the most widely known and easily accessible interviews is described in this section. The Vineland Adaptive Behavior Scales–Interview Edition (Sparrow et al. 1984) is a semistructured interview measure of personal and social skills from birth to adulthood. This well-known instrument provides T-scores, age equivalents, and national percentile rankings in the domains of Communication, Daily Living Skills, Socialization Skills, and Motor Skills. Supplemental norms are available for individuals with disabilities. The K-SADS (Chambers et al. 1985) mentioned earlier in this chapter has been widely used as a research and clinical assessment measure for both parents and children. There are currently several K-SADS versions, all of which are semistructured integrated parent–child interviews. Data from parents and children are recorded on a common answer sheet by a single interviewer. The K-SADS-PL (Kaufman et al. 1997), also mentioned previously, provides for the diagnosis of PTSD symptoms, although the training necessary for its administration may preclude it from clinical use. The Anxiety Disorders Interview Schedule for DSM-IV Child Version (Albano and Silverman 1996) is a semistructured interview measure with companion versions for the parent and child. The interview format was designed to help diagnose disorders, including PTSD, in which anxiety is the prominent feature. The Child Interview Schedule provides a "Feelings Thermometer," a visual cue designed to help children report feelings of distress. It is a clinician-friendly measure that uses an icon system for more accurate application of DSM-IV criteria.

Several parent-report inventories are available, are widely used in the clinical assessment of emotional and behavioral disorders, and are particularly applicable for assessing PTSD. The Achenbach Child Behavior Checklist (CBCL; Achenbach and Edelbrock 1983) has been used extensively in PTSD research and clinical applications as a checklist measure of internalizing and externalizing behaviors. The utility of the CBCL is enhanced by the use of its "family" of measures, the Youth Self Report inventory (YSR; Achenbach and Edelbrock 1987) and the Teacher Report version. The report form also provides a section where parents can describe their beliefs about their child's academic and social functioning as well as concerns about emotional functioning. A Spanish version is also available. A more extensive parent-report inventory of behavior and personality functioning is provided by the PIC, mentioned earlier in the chapter, which is administered as a short (280 items) or long (427 items) true/false inventory. It yields personality factor scales, clinical scales, and, perhaps most important, validity scales. The PIC has sometimes been referred to as a "kiddie MMPI" and was originally developed by members of the MMPI authorship team. Although the PIC is not used for diagnosing PTSD specifically, it is one of the most robust and widely used personality inventories. Its validity scales (based on parent as informant) can be useful in determining underreporting of symptoms, exaggeration, and defensive approach to the test.

Clinical Interview of Children and Adolescents

Clinical interviewing should be initially facilitated through both informal questions and observation. Engaging children in the interview process may be difficult because avoidance behaviors, denial, numbing, and traumatic amnesia are common manifestations in children with PTSD (Terr 1994). With very young children, an informal play and conversation period is recommended to make them feel at ease. Roleplay with dolls or small human figures is an effective and well-known method of generating a child's report of a traumatic event (Koocher et al. 1995). Besides structured play as an interview procedure, observing the child in free play may provide the clinician with the chance to observe repetitive themes about the event.

As many pediatric specialists know, drawing tasks are an effective and nonthreatening way to initiate the evaluation with young children (Webb 1991). The characters, scenes, and themes they depict can facilitate more formal interviewing. In addition to asking children to describe their events as stories, Terr (1996) recommends asking them to draw pictures of the event or "what brings them to the office." Another strategy is to ask children to draw a timeline of their lives with key events depicted in pictures along a line drawn by the interviewer. What is omitted—as well as what is depicted in the drawings, roleplay, or story—is significant and may yield additional diagnostic information. Behaviors observed while the child is describing the drawings are equally important (Terr 1996). In addition to their use as an expressive and reporting modality, drawing tests are used to identify personality characteristics in response to a trauma and/or abuse that are not easily assessed by self-report measures (Blain et al. 1981). The most well-known projective drawing test is the House-Tree-Person test developed and popularized by Buck (1948). Today, quantitative scoring systems are available for interpreting the House-Tree-Person test and Draw-A-Person projective techniques (Van Hutton 1994). These tests have been used extensively in assessing symptoms of physical and sexual abuse (Van Hutton 1994).

Although interviewing a child about the details of a traumatic experience may intuitively raise concerns of retraumatization, at least one study indicates that an initial PTSD screening and/or interview conducted shortly after the trauma may serve to lessen future PTSD symptoms and promote recovery (Nader et al. 1990). Pynoos and Eth (1986) noted that the interview can be conducted shortly after the trauma, even with very young children. They present a comprehensive model for interviewing young children that includes an introduction, a drawing and storytelling exercise to elicit material about the trauma, elaboration of the story, linking the story or drawing to some aspect of the trauma, and then an elaboration and working through of the trauma. In the final stage of the interview, the child reviews and summarizes the session and links the current problems to the trauma. Finally, the child is encouraged to talk about the interview, both helpful aspects and upsetting aspects. This is only a summary of the interview described by Pynoos and Eth (1986); therefore, we recommend that the reader refer to the original article for specific details.

Beyond the clinical diagnostic interview that is adapted to assess for PTSD symptoms, there are multiple semistructured clinical interviews in addition to those previously reviewed that can be used to fully assess the nature and extent of current PTSD symptoms. One of the oldest semistructured interview measures is the Children's Depression Rating Scale–Revised (CDRS-R; Poznanski et al. 1985), which has been used extensively for clinical and research purposes in both normal patients and depressed patients. The CDRS-R is easy to administer with brief training. A scoring system based on number and intensity of symptoms indicates the severity of depression. Moreover, the CDRS-R can provide an effective framework for interviewing children about emotional functioning in general as well as symptoms characteristic of PTSD. The Diagnostic Interview for Children and Adolescents–Revised (Reich et al. 1991) and the Diagnostic Interview Schedule for Children–Supplemental PTSD Module (Shaffer et al. 2000) have been used over the past several years in research as well as clinical settings. A more recently developed measure is the Interview Schedule for Children and Adolescents (Sherrill and Kovacs 2000), a structured interview for psychiatric and medical populations that yields symptom ratings relevant to PTSD.

Regardless of the specific instrument used, the structured clinical interview is a valuable tool in clinical assessment. However, as Peterson (1993) noted, no instrument is foolproof and therefore should never substitute for clinical acumen and a solid knowledge of diagnostic criteria.

Cognitive Assessment

As noted earlier, the assessment and evaluation of PTSD in children and adolescents must be considered within a developmental context, because PTSD has a chronic course that can derail a child from his or her developmental track. Regressive behaviors, diminished attention, and memory problems have been observed in children and adolescents (Pelcovitz et al. 1996; Perrin et al. 2000; Pfefferbaum 1997). Therefore, cognitive assessment— including assessment of intelligence, memory, language, and executive functioning—should be considered an integral part of a PTSD evaluation. The rationale for including cognitive assessment in an evaluation for PTSD is to a) determine the child's current level of intellectual functioning, memory, developmental stage, and academic functioning; b) analyze the child's measured functional abilities in relation to developmental stage; and c) differentiate between developmental and cognitive influences in the diagnosis of PTSD. Most important, including cognitive assessment in the evaluation process provides the clinician with critical objective data about the child's or adolescent's overall level of functioning.

It is recommended that psychiatrists work with licensed child psychologists or neuropsychologists with expertise in the assessment of children and adolescents. Generally, the role of the neuropsychologist in PTSD evaluations is to develop an assessment battery, administer the instruments, score and interpret the results, and provide feedback. Both objective measures (e.g., tests of intelligence, achievement, language, and memory) and subjective or projective measures (e.g., emotional and personality inventories) are then interpreted within the context of the individual and the referral question. Recommendations for psychosocial and educational interventions are also included in feedback sessions.

Cognitive assessment, as a component of a PTSD evaluation, involves a comprehensive battery of tests that includes standardized measures of intelligence, language, attention, visual spatial abilities, and memory. There are several standardized measures of intelligence, including screening instruments for intellectual functioning and measures for all age groups. General measures of intelligence, such as the Wechsler Intelligence Scale for Children–Third Edition (Wechsler 1991) yield IQ scores on the verbal and nonverbal domains. Standardized measures of general memory functioning as well as measures of working memory, visual memory, and auditory memory should be used in the evaluation of PTSD, given the noted impact of PTSD on memory in particular (Moradi et al. 1999). Various instruments and interactive tests have been developed for assessing executive functioning in children. These measures focus on attention, working memory, cognitive flexibility, inductive reasoning, and resistance to interference. Although a review of cognitive measures in assessment is beyond the scope of this chapter, the reader is encouraged to include a variety of standardized cognitive functioning, memory, and achievement measures in the PTSD evaluation.

In school-age children and adolescents, a PTSD evaluation should include at least a screening assessment of academic achievement. The clinician is advised not to rely exclusively on prior psychoeducational testing administered by the child's school. Rather, prior educational testing should be used as supportive data and background information with which to compare current test results.

Emotional Functioning

For school-aged children and adolescents, several self-report inventories exist that assess PTSD symptoms and more comprehensive aspects of the disorder. Several self-report and semi-structured interview measures, discussed earlier in this chapter, have been used in the assessment of PTSD in children and adolescents. Emotional and personality functioning can be assessed using self-report measures developed specifically for determining whether symptoms meet DSM-IV criteria for PTSD. By contrast, clinicians can administer well-known, standardized measures of depression, anxiety, and personality that, when results are combined, yield a symptom profile consistent with the DSM-IV diagnostic criteria for PTSD.

Self-Report Measures

Bernstein et al. (1994) developed the Childhood Trauma Questionnaire, a self-report inventory that has been used with adolescents who experienced traumatic events as children. This inventory is particularly sensitive to identifying symptoms of PTSD relevant to physical and sexual abuse cases. As mentioned previously, the TSCC (Briere 1996a, 1996b) is also extremely useful for assessing PTSD and related symptoms in children because of its substantial normative sample and inclusion of validity scales. One of the most widely used and enduring measures is the Impact of Events Scale (IES; Horowitz et al. 1979), which was originally developed for adults but has been adapted for clinical and research purposes in the diagnosis of PTSD in children and adolescents (Yule and Udwin 1991; Yule and Williams 1990).

There are several non–PTSD-specific self-report measures that have been extensively used in the research and clinical evaluation of PTSD-related symptoms. Some of the best-known and easily accessible include The Child Depression Inventory (CDI; Kovacs 1992), the Reynolds Adolscent Depression Scale (Reynolds 1987), and the Revised Children's Manifest Anxiety Scale (RCMAS; Reynolds and Richmond 1978), for which a Spanish-language version is also available. Measures to assess for dissociation, such as the Adolescent Dissociative Experiences Scale (A-DES; Armstrong et al. 1997) or the Child Dissociative Checklist (CDC; Putnam 1994) should also be included in any battery assessing PTSD.

Assessment of emotional and personality functioning in adolescents at risk for PTSD should, if possible, include the MMPI-A (Butcher et al. 1992), a 468-item self-report inventory developed for use in adolescents ages 14–18. The MMPI-A yields scores on content scales, supplementary scales, and validity scales and provides a robust measure of affective symptoms and aspects of personality functioning. A computerized interpretive scoring system for the MMPI-A is available that provides indices sensitive to symptoms (e.g., anxiety, expression, social discomfort, and repression) and treatment indications.

Projective Techniques

The use of projective measures in the evaluation of children and adolescents for PTSD is important for several reasons. First, children may have difficulty directly expressing their feelings of distress (Pynoos and Eth 1986; Terr 1994). Second, projective measures provide an unstructured platform on which both conscious and unconscious aspects of emotional functioning can be assessed. Projective measures can be useful in assessing a child's coping style, gaining a greater sense of the child's pervasive fears or anxieties, and exploring the themes about the trauma that influence the child's sense of self in relationship to others. Projective measures facilitate the assessment of personality and emotional functioning by giving the child freedom to create his or her own structure and meaning from ambiguous stimuli. Projective measures should be administered only by a qualified professional who is well trained in their administration, scoring, and interpretation because these measures are extremely dependent on the skill of the administrator. With this in mind, a few of the well-known and most child-friendly projective measures are discussed below.

The Rorschach Inkblot Test (Rorschach 1921/1942) is the most popular projective measure among clinicians and has a long history of use in the evaluation of psychologic disorders in children (Exner and Weiner 1995; Weiner 1996). Holaday et al. (1992) described the use of the Rorschach test specifically in assessing traumatized children. The Rorschach test can be most useful in assessing personality organization and, in children, the developmental capacity for reality testing and integration of affect.

Although several scoring systems have been developed over several decades, the comprehensive system developed by Exner (1993) represents the most standardized method of scoring and interpretation. The Children's Apperception Test (CAT; Bellak and Bellak 1998) is the most well-known projective measure for young children. It is similar in many respects to the Thematic Apperception Test (TAT) developed by Murray (1943). The CAT is recommended for use in children ages 3–10 years and features pictures of animals that are often in tension-filled situations. As part of the test, the child is asked to tell a story about the picture with a beginning, a middle, and a conclusion. The use of animals is based on the theory that young children may identify more easily with animals rather than human figures. A "human figure" version of the CAT, the CAT–H, is also published for use with older children and in research. The Roberts Apperception Test for Children (RATC; Roberts and McArthur 1982) is a projective test that provides an objective scoring system and norms. The RATC stimuli, like those used in the CAT and TAT, are pictures of children in various familial and social situations. Responses are scored based on the presence or absence of specific characteristics. The RATC measures adaptive and maladaptive functioning and yields T-scores on clinical scales such as Reliance on Others, Anxiety, Depression, Rejection, Unresolved Problems, and Resolution.

Another type of projective measure is the sentence completion test. The Rotter Incomplete Sentence Blank (Rotter and Rafferty 1950) is most likely the best-known test of its kind. A newer version, the Sentence Completion Series (SCS; Brown and Unger 1992) is available in forms for use in the clinical assessment of adolescents. Briefly, sentence completion tests consist of 40–50 items composed of incomplete sentences or "sentence stems." The child or adolescent completes the sentence to express his or her true feelings. Although manual-based scoring systems are available, most often a clinical approach to sentence analysis is used. The Children's Self-Report and Projective Inventory (CSRPI; Ziffer and Shapiro 1992) provides self-report, sentence completion, and projective measures in one kit. The CSRPI components can be used in their entirety or individually for the assessment of emotional functioning.

Conclusions

PTSD in children is a complex, dynamic diagnostic entity that can potentially affect all aspects of a child's emotional, developmental, and cognitive functioning. Therefore, its assessment in the clinical, as opposed to research, setting requires an equally varied approach that assesses all potentially affected domains. By assessing a broad domain of psychologic and cognitive functioning, the clinician can develop a more complete diagnostic picture, even when initial resistance is met in the interview process or limited information is available from the patient. For example, a child who has been exposed to trauma may deny or underreport symptoms in a face-to-face interview. However, an interview with his or her parents may reveal a new onset of night terrors and decreased interaction with peers. Cognitive testing may indicate decreased attention and memory functioning as compared with other aspects of cognition, and conversations with teachers may indicate poorer school performance than would be expected based on intellectual and academic testing. The inclusion of a measure with validity scales might indicate that the child is not admitting to commonly endorsed behaviors. Projective measures may uncover themes of trauma and loss that would not otherwise be revealed. Together, these results begin to paint a picture that is not inconsistent with PTSD and that will aid the clinician in ruling out other possible diagnoses.

Test results, however, must never be interpreted in isolation or considered outside the total context of the history and presenting problem of the individual being assessed, for as one prominent neuropsychologist has noted, "a test result is not a diagnosis." This should be the mantra of all professionals whose duties involve assessment and diagnosis. No test is foolproof, no matter how well validated, and tests can only be considered an aid to the clinician in making a diagnosis. They are not a substitute for face-to-face time with the patient or for well-developed diagnostic skills and clinical reasoning. However, when used properly, comprehensive assessment is a benefit to clinician and patient alike.

References

Achenbach T, Edelbrock C: Manual for the Child Behavior Checklist and Revised Child Behavior Profile. Burlington, VT, University of Vermont Department of Psychiatry, 1983

Achenbach T, Edelbrock C: Manual for the Youth Self-Report and Profile. Burlington, VT, University of Vermont Department of Psychiatry, 1987

Albano AM, Silverman W: Anxiety Disorders Interview Schedule for DSM-IV Child Version. San Antonio, TX, Psychological Corporation, 1996

American Psychiatric Association: Diagnostic and Statistical Manual of Mental Disorders, 3rd Edition. Washington, DC, American Psychiatric Association, 1980

American Psychiatric Association: Diagnostic and Statistical Manual of Mental Disorders, 3rd Edition Revised. Washington, DC, American Psychiatric Association, 1987

American Psychiatric Association: Diagnostic and Statistical Manual of Mental Disorders, 4th Edition. Washington, DC, American Psychiatric Association, 1994

Angold A, Pendergast M, Cox M, et al: The Child and Adolescent Psychiatric Assessment. Psychol Med 25:739–753, 1995

Armstrong J, Putnam FW, Carlson E, et al: Development and validation of a measure of adolescent dissociation: The Adolescent Dissociative Experiences Scale. J Nerv Ment Dis 185:491–497, 1997

Bellak L, Bellak S: Children's Apperception Test, Ninth Revised Edition. Larchmont, NY, C.P.S. Inc, 1998

Bernstein DP, Fink L, Handelsman L, et al: Initial reliability and validity of a new retrospective measure of child abuse and neglect. Am J Psychiatry 151:1132–1136, 1994

Blain GH, Bergner RM, Lewis ML, et al: The use of objectively scorable House-Tree-Person indicators to establish child abuse. J Clin Psychol 37:667–673, 1981

Briere J: Trauma Symptom Checklist for Children (TSCC). Odessa, FL, Psychological Assessment Resources, 1996a

Briere J: Trauma Symptom Checklist for Children (TSCC) Professional Manual. Odessa, FL, Psychological Assessment Resources, 1996b

Brown LH, Unger AM: Sentence Completion Series (SCS). Odessa, FL, Psychological Assessment Resources, 1992

Buck JN: The H-T-P technique: a qualitative and quantitative scoring manual. J Clin Psychol 4:317–396, 1948

Butcher JN, Williams CL, Graham JR, et al: MMPI-A: Manual for Administration, Scoring and Interpretation. Minneapolis, MN, University of Minnesota Press, 1992

Carlson EB: Trauma Assessments: A Clinician's Guide. New York, Guilford, 1997

Chambers W, Puig-Antich J, Hirsch M, et al: The assessment of affective disorders in children and adolescents by semi-structured interview: test–retest reliability of the Schedule for Affective Disorders and Schizophrenia for School-Age Children, Present Episode version. Arch Gen Psychiatry 42:696–702, 1985

Cohen JA, American Academy of Child and Adolescent Psychiatry Work Group on Quality Issues: Practice parameters for the assessment and treatment of children and adolescents with posttraumatic stress disorder. J Am Acad Child Adolesc Psychiatry 37(suppl):4S–26S, 1998

Costello EJ, Angold A, March JS, et al: Life events and post-traumatic stress: the development of a new measure for children and adolescents. Psychol Med 28:1275–1288, 1998

Earls F, Smith E, Reich W, et al: Investigating psychopathological consequences of a disaster in children: a pilot study incorporating a structured diagnostic interview. J Am Acad Child Adolesc Psychiatry 27:90–95, 1988

Exner JE: The Rorschach: A Comprehensive System, Vol 1: Basic Foundations, 3rd Edition. New York, Wiley, 1993

Exner JE, Weiner IB: The Rorschach: A Comprehensive System, Vol 3: Assessment of Children and Adolescents, 2nd Edition. New York, Wiley, 1995

Frederick C: Children traumatized by catastrophic situations, in Post-Traumatic Stress Disorder in Children. Edited by Eth S, Pynoos RS. Washington, DC, American Psychiatric Press, 1985, pp 73–99

Frederick C, Pynoos R, Nader K: Childhood PTSD Reaction Index (CPTS-RI), 1992. Available on request from Frederick and Pynoos, 760 Westwood Plaza, Los Angeles, CA 90024 or Nader, P.O. Box 2251, Laguna Hills, CA 92654

Holaday M, Armsworth MW, Swank PR, et al: Rorschach responding in traumatized children and adolescents. J Trauma Stress 5:119–129, 1992

Horowitz M, Wilner N, Alvarez W: Impact of Events Scale: a measure of subjective stress. Psychosom Med 41:209–218, 1979

Kaufman J, Birmaher B, Brent D, et al: Schedule for Affective Disorders and Schizophrenia for School-Age Children–Present and Lifetime Version (K-SADS-PL): initial reliability and validity data. J Am Acad Child Adolesc Psychiatry 36:980–988, 1997

Koocher GP, Goodman GS, White S, et al: Psychological science and the use of anatomically detailed dolls in child sexual abuse assessments: final report of the American Psychological Association Anatomical Doll Task Force. Psychol Bull 118:199–222, 1995

Kovacs M: Children's Depression Inventory. North Tonawanda, NY, Multi-Health Systems, 1992

McFarlane AC: Family functioning and overprotection following a natural disaster: the longitudinal effects of post-traumatic morbidity. Aust N Z J Psychiatry 21:210–218, 1987

McNally RJ: Assessment of posttraumatic stress disorder in children. Psychological Assessment 3:531–537, 1991

Moradi AR, Neshat Doost HT, Taghavi MR, et al: Everyday memory deficits in children and adolescents with PTSD: performance on the Rivermead Behavioural Memory Test. J Child Psychol Psychiatry 40:357–361, 1999

Murray HA: Explorations in Personality. New York, Oxford University Press, 1943

Nader KO: Assessing traumatic experience in children, in Assessing Psychological Trauma and PTSD. Edited by Wilson JP, Keane TM. New York, Guilford, 1997, pp 291–348

Nader K, Pynoos R: School disaster: planning and initial interventions. Journal of Social Behavior and Personality 8:299–320, 1993

Nader K, Pynoos R, Fairbanks L, et al: Children's PTSD reactions one year after a sniper attack at their school. Am J Psychiatry 147:1526–1530, 1990

Nader KO, Newman E, Weathers FW, et al: Clinician Administered PTSD Scale for Children and Adolescents for DSM-IV (CAPS-CA). Lebanon, NH, The Hitchcock Foundation, 1998

Neugebauer R, Wasserman GA, Fisher PW, et al: Darryl, a cartoon-based measure of cardinal posttraumatic stress symptoms in school-age children. Am J Public Health 89:758–761, 1999

Newman CJ: Children of disaster: clinical observations at Buffalo Creek. Am J Psychiatry 133:306–312, 1976

Newman E, McMackin RA, Morrisey C, et al: PTSD among incarcerated male adolescents at secure juvenile treatment facilities (1998). Unpublished raw data as reported in Saigh PA, Yasik AE, Oberfield RA, et al: The Children's PTSD Inventory: development and reliability. J Trauma Stress 13:369–380, 2000

Pelcovitz D, Kaplan S: Post-traumatic stress disorder in children and adolescents. Child and Adolescent Psychiatric Clinics of North America 5:449–496, 1996

Pelcovitz D, Kaplan S, Goldenberg B, et al: Post-traumatic stress disorder in physically abused adolescents. J Am Acad Child Adolesc Psychiatry 33:305–312, 1994

Perrin S, Smith P, Yule W: Practitioner review: the assessment and treatment of post-traumatic stress disorder in children and adolescents. Journal of Child Psychology and Psychiatry 41:277–289, 2000

Peterson G: Limitations of structural interviews. J Am Acad Child Adolesc Psychiatry 32:469, 1993

Pfefferbaum B: Posttraumatic stress disorder in children: a review of the past 10 years. J Am Acad Child Adolesc Psychiatry 36:1503–1511, 1997

Poznanski EO, Freeman LN, Mokros HB et al: Children's Depression Rating Scale–Revised. Psychopharmacol Bull 4:979–989, 1985

Putnam FW: Child Dissociative Checklist, 1994. Available on request from the author, Unit of Developmental Traumatology, NIMH, Building 15K, 9000 Rockville Pike, Bethesda, MD 20892

Pynoos RS, Eth S: Children traumatized by witnessing acts of personal violence: homicide, rape, or suicide behavior, in Post-Traumatic Stress Disorder in Children. Edited by Eth S, Pynoos RS. Washington, DC, American Psychiatric Press, 1985, pp 17–43

Pynoos RS, Eth S: Witness to violence: the child interview. J Am Acad Child Adolesc Psychiatry 25:306–319, 1986

Pynoos RS, Frederick, C, Nader K, et al: Life threat and posttraumatic stress in school-age children. Arch Gen Psychiatry 44:1057–1063, 1987

Reich W, Shayka JJ, Taibleson C: Diagnostic Interview for Children and Adolescents (DICA). St. Louis, MO, Washington University, 1991

Reynolds CR: Reynolds Adolescent Depression Scale (RADS). Odessa, FL, Psychological Assessment Resources, 1987

Reynolds CR, Richmond BO: What I think and feel: a revised measure of children's manifest anxiety. J Abnorm Child Psychol 6:271–280, 1978

Roberts GE, McArthur DS: Roberts Apperception Test for Children. Los Angeles, CA, Western Psychological Services, 1982

Rorschach H: Psychodiagnostics: a diagnostic test based on perception (1921). New York, Grune & Stratton, 1942

Rotter JB, Rafferty JE: The Manual for the Rotter Incomplete Sentences Blank. New York, Psychological Corporation, 1950

Ruggiero KJ, McLeer SV: PTSD scale of the Child Behavior Checklist: concurrent and discriminant validity with non-clinic-referred sexually abused children. J Trauma Stress 13:287–299, 2000

Saigh PA, Yasik AE, Oberfield RA, et al: The Children's PTSD Inventory: development and reliability. J Trauma Stress 13:369–380, 2000

Sattler JM: Clinical and Forensic Interviewing of Children and Families: Guidelines for the Mental Health, Education, Pediatric, and Child Maltreatment Fields. San Diego, CA, Sattler, 1997

Shaffer D, Fisher P, Lucas CP, et al: NIMH Diagnostic Interview Schedule for Children Version IV (NIMH DISC-IV): description, differences from previous versions, and reliability of some common diagnoses. J Am Acad Child Adolesc Psychiatry 39:28–38, 2000

Sherrill JT, Kovacs M: Interview schedule for children and adolescents (ISCA). J Am Acad Child Adolesc Psychiatry 39:67–75, 2000

Sparrow SS, Balla DA, Ciccheti DV: Vineland Adaptive Behavior Scales. Circle Pines, MN, American Guidance Service Inc., 1984

Terr LC: Childhood traumas: an outline and overview. Am J Psychiatry 148:10–20, 1991

Terr LC: Unchained memories: true stories of traumatic memories lost and found. New York, Basic Books, 1994

Terr LC: Acute responses to external events and posttraumatic stress disorder, in Child and Adolescent Psychiatry: A Comprehensive Textbook, 2nd Edition. Edited by Lewis M. New Haven, CT, Williams & Wilkins, 1996, pp 753–801

Van Hutton V: H-T-P/D-A-P as measures of abuse in children: a quantitative scoring system. Odessa, FL, Psychological Assessment Resources, 1994

Webb NB: Play Therapy with Children in Crisis: A Casebook for Practitioners. New York, Guilford, 1991

Wechsler D: Wechsler Intelligence Scale for Children–Third Edition. San Antonio, TX, The Psychological Corporation, 1991

Weiner IB: Some observations on the validity of the Rorschach Inkblot Method. Psychological Assessment 8:206–213, 1996

Wirt RD, Lachar D, Klinedinst JK, et al: Multidimensional description of child personality: a manual for the Personality Inventory for Children, Revised. Los Angeles, CA, Western Psychological Services, 1990

Yehuda R, McFarlane AC: Conflict between current knowledge about posttraumatic stress disorder and its original conceptual basis. Am J Psychiatry 152:1705–1713, 1995

Yule W, Udwin O: Screening child survivors for post-traumatic stress disorders: Experiences from the "Jupiter" sinking. Br J Clin Psychol 30:131–138, 1991

Yule W, Williams R: Post-traumatic stress reactions in children. J Trauma Stress 3:279–295, 1990

Ziffer RL, Shapiro LE: Children's Self-Report and Projective Inventory (CSPRI). Los Angeles, CA, Psychological Assessment Service, 1992

Chapter 2

Forensic Aspects of PTSD in Children and Adolescents

James E. Rosenberg, M.D.

Introduction

Stone (1993) once wrote, "No diagnosis in the history of American psychiatry has had a more dramatic and pervasive impact on law and social justice than post-traumatic stress disorder" (p. 23). Nowhere do these words ring more true than in the field of child and adolescent forensic psychiatry.

The study of posttraumatic stress disorder (PTSD) in children and adolescents is a relatively new discipline—one that is exploding with a variety of important developments that can potentially help or hinder the forensic psychiatrist. Experts must realistically assess their own qualifications for undertaking such evaluations and must be properly attuned to the shortcomings and complexities inherent in evaluating whether a child or teenager qualifies for a diagnosis of PTSD. Embedded within this process is an appreciation for the research and controversy surrounding the reliability of child victim testimony and of recovered memories in adulthood, whether recovered in the psychiatrist's office or the courtroom.

The accepted diagnostic terms and criteria for the psychologic sequelae of trauma have undergone considerable evolution over the past 50 years. Before the Vietnam War and the attendant advances in neuroscience, adult trauma victims were evaluated and treated primarily within a Freudian paradigm (Boehnlein 1989). The original Diagnostic and Statistical Manual (DSM), published by the American Psychiatric Association (APA) in 1952, referred to the emotional response to trauma as a *gross stress reaction*. In 1968, the DSM-II was released, which used the appellation *transient situational disturbance* (American Psychiatric Association 1968; Brett et al. 1988).

The term *posttraumatic stress disorder* was introduced in 1980 with the publication of DSM-III (American Psychiatric Association 1980). This was indeed a turning point in the history of PTSD in psychiatry. In addition to ushering the acronym *PTSD* into common diagnostic usage, DSM-III introduced the concept of a chronic version of posttraumatic anxiety and dropped preexisting psychopathology as an exclusion. Furthermore, the U.S. Department of Veterans Affairs accepted the DSM-III diagnosis of PTSD, delayed type, allowing veterans for the first time since World War I to apply for service-connected disability 1 year or more after their periods of military service had expired. There was no specific reference to child trauma in the PTSD section until DSM-III-R (American Psychiatric Association 1987). In DSM-IV (American Psychiatric Association 1994), acute stress disorder was introduced as an early onset alternative to acute PTSD with an emphasis on dissociative symptoms.

Special consideration for child trauma and its consequences began with a series of case studies dating back to the mid-1970s, including Newman's 1976 report on the Buffalo Creek disaster and Terr's (1979) landmark paper on the Chowchilla kidnapping incident.

Diagnosis

As discussed in DSM-IV, the diagnosis of PTSD requires that the patient experience a threshold traumatic event followed by a triad of reexperiencing, avoidance and numbing, and hyperarousal symptoms. With regard to what qualifies as a traumatic event (i.e., Criterion A), "the person experienced, witnessed, or was confronted with...actual or threatened death or serious injury, or a threat to the physical integrity of self or others...the person's response involved intense fear, helplessness, or horror" (DSM-IV-TR, p. 467). In children, this response may manifest as disorganized behavior or agitation.

Pynoos et al. (1996) pointed out that traumatic stress may continue after the explicit violence or other crisis has passed (e.g., staying by an injured or dead family member until help arrives) and that the stress may be "multilayered":

> In traumatic situations, the experience of external threat involves an estimation of the extreme magnitude of the threat, the unavailability or ineffectiveness of contemplated or actual protective actions by self or others, and the experience of physical helplessness at irreversible traumatic moments. The experience of internal threat includes a sense of inability to tolerate the affective responses and physiological reactions, as well as a sense of catastrophic personal consequence. (p. 338)

Thus, a personal threat to a child may be accompanied by fear for the safety of a loved one and other features that only heighten the trauma.

DSM-IV Criterion B for PTSD requires that the individual reexperience the traumatic event in one or more of several possible ways: recurrent, intrusive memories; nightmares; acting or feeling as though the traumatic event is happening again, such as in hallucinations or flashbacks; intense psychologic distress at exposure to trauma-related cues; and psychophysiologic reactivity to such cues. Presentation may have important differences in younger children, whereas symptoms become more like those of adults in older children and teenagers. In place of explicit, intrusive memories, traumatized children may engage in joyless, repetitive play that symbolizes the trauma in part or as a whole. Incident-specific nightmares may be replaced with frightening dreams of monsters or more general content involving dangers and threats. Reenactment behaviors may occur that are akin to flashbacks in adults.

Criterion C involves the presence of three or more avoidance and numbing symptoms from a total list of seven: 1) cognitive avoidance behaviors, such as refusing to discuss the event; 2) situational avoidance, (e.g., steering clear of places, people, or other things that trigger posttraumatic memories); 3) some degree of psychogenic amnesia; 4) loss of interest or pleasure in significant activities; 5) emotional isolation or numbing from others; 6) lack of emotional range; and 7) a sense of a foreshortened future.

Many of these items can be difficult to elicit in the child interview and require a greater reliance on outside sources of information such as parents, teachers, or relatives. Children's pessimism about the future may take the form of not expecting to reach adulthood or other later developmental milestones. They may also engage in omen formation—thoughts and feelings of being able to predict future adverse events.

Finally, Criterion D pertains to autonomic hyperarousal symptoms. The trauma victim is required to have two or more of the following: sleep disturbance, irritability or angry outbursts, concentration problems, excessive vigilance, and/or an increased startle reaction to environmental stimuli. In addition, children may exhibit or complain of various physical ailments (American Psychiatric Association 2000).

Differential diagnoses include acute stress disorder, adjustment disorder, attention-deficit/hyperactivity disorder (ADHD), and other anxiety disorders. The severity of the stressor, its relevance to the onset and course of the patient's symptoms, and the timing, breadth, and natural history of those symptoms are all pertinent to the assessment process.

Terr (1991) formulated two different types of PTSD based on the frequency and duration of the trauma. In Type I traumas, in which the child experiences a single traumatic event such as an accidental injury, the classic triad of reexperiencing, avoidance and numbing, and hyperarousal symptoms potentially follows. Detailed memories, omen formation, and perceptual disturbances occur. In contrast, in Type II traumas, in which the child experiences repetitive or chronic traumatic experiences such as repeated sexual abuse over a period of years, a different profile of symptoms develops. Presentation is more one of denial, dissociative symptoms, emotional numbing, and anger. Some victims can also experience a hybrid of Type I and II features (Terr 1991).

Blank (1993) outlined the extraordinary variability in the onset and course of PTSD. His review of the PTSD literature indicated that, in addition to acute, chronic, and delayed-type forms, PTSD can be intermittent or recurrent. The relative proportions of reexperiencing, avoidance and numbing, and hyperarousal symptoms vary with the individual and the trauma experience and fluctuate over time for a particular case. The severity and other characteristics of PTSD only partially correlate with the severity, proximity, and duration of the traumatic event.

The variability of the natural history of PTSD is underscored by the research on the association between acute stress disorder and PTSD. Using a study group of motor vehicle accident victims, the authors assessed the incidence of acute stress disorder and then the percentage of subjects who qualified for PTSD 2 years after the trauma (Harvey and Bryant 1999). Thirteen percent of the victims met diagnostic criteria for acute stress disorder, and another 21% had a subsyndromal version. Interestingly, at 2 years posttrauma, 63% of the subjects who had initially met diagnostic criteria for acute stress disorder now qualified for PTSD, whereas 70% of those who had had subsyndromal acute stress disorder had PTSD. Another 13% who never met criteria for either acute stress disorder category had also developed PTSD. Thus, this study suggests that acute stress disorder must not be viewed as a necessary precursor to PTSD because individuals with subsyndromal acute stress disorder and those with no stress disorder were still at significant risk of developing PTSD.

The differential diagnosis between ADHD and PTSD is important because of the seeming overlap of symptoms between these disorders and their relative frequencies in pediatric populations. For example, in a study comparing sexually abused and non–sexually abused children who were referred to a psychiatric clinic, McLeer et al. (1994) found that, in both groups, ADHD was the most prevalent diagnosis. However, 42.3% of the abused children met diagnostic criteria for PTSD compared with only 8.7% of the nonabused children.

The impulsivity, hyperactivity, and interpersonal difficulties encountered in ADHD could be misidentified as hyperarousal symptoms in PTSD, or vice versa (Weinstein et al. 2000). Furthermore, treatment for the two disorders is very different; misdiagnosis will likely lead to medication therapy that is either ineffective or actually detrimental. Stimulant medications, the first-line treatment for ADHD, would potentially aggravate a host of symptoms in PTSD, including autonomic hyperactivity and sleep difficulties. Given the relative prevalence of both disorders, PTSD should be contemplated in cases suggestive of child trauma before a premature or sole diagnosis of ADHD is reached in the inattentive, impulsive, easily agitated child.

Two interesting scenarios arise in the diagnosis of stress-related anxiety disorders (McNally and Saigh 1993). First, if the patient develops the triad of PTSD symptoms—reexperiencing phenomena, avoidance and numbing, and hyperarousal—in response to a nontraumatic or subthreshold stressor, the appropriate diagnosis is adjustment disorder or anxiety disorder not otherwise specified. The former diagnosis is preferable to the latter because it is less vague and generic and at least provides the etiologic element of a stressor. The second scenario involves the patient who, in response to an emotional trauma, as defined under DSM-IV Criterion A for PTSD, develops only fear and avoidance symptoms. The appropriate diagnosis is specific phobia. This diagnosis, unlike PTSD or adjustment disorder, is independent of etiology.

Epidemiology

Lifetime prevalence of PTSD is estimated from community-based studies to be 8% (American Psychiatric Association 2000). Kessler et al. (1999) presented the results of the National Comorbidity Study, which included 8,098 respondents. Of these, 60.7% of men and 51.2% of women reported having experienced at least one traumatic event in their lifetimes. Most experienced two or more traumas. The risk of developing PTSD varied with the type of trauma. The three types of traumas that were most likely to cause PTSD—rape, childhood physical abuse, and childhood neglect—had occurred more commonly in women.

Deykin (1999) pointed out how differences in data collection can influence the reported prevalence of PTSD. Although the Epidemiologic Catchment Area study estimated the prevalence of the disorder at about 1%, the National Comorbidity Study, conducted over several years in the early 1990s, artificially raised the rate with its estimate of 7.8% because data were collected from a subpopulation in which all individuals already had some sort of mental disorder.

Epidemiologic studies have demonstrated a high rate of co-morbidity of other psychiatric disorders with PTSD in adults. Most patients have at least one other disorder, and a significant percentage have three or more. The greatest rates of comorbidity with PTSD were seen in depressive, substance use, and anxiety disorders (Brady et al. 2000).

Genetics

As noted in DSM-IV, there is evidence of a heritable component to the transmission of PTSD. For example, using the Vietnam Era Twin Registry and controlling for combat exposure, True and Lyons (1999) studied the relative contributions of genetic and environmental factors in the genesis of various PTSD symptoms. In general, genetic predisposition accounted for about 30% of the liability for developing a particular reexperiencing, avoidance and numbing, and hyperarousal symptom as compared with environmental factors. The one exception was intrusive, unpleasant memories, which appeared to carry only about a 10% genetic liability.

Risk Factors in Various Settings

Several factors in addition to the trauma itself can affect whether an event results in PTSD, including the characteristics of the traumatic experience, the make-up of the victim, the environment, and the availability of social and family support (Deykin 1999). Deykin (1999), in a review of the literature, found a consensus that the rate of PTSD is higher in females than males, even when one controls for rape.

In her review of the literature on gender effects in the genesis of PTSD, Pfefferbaum (1997) found mixed results. Some studies found a higher rate of symptom development in girls, others reported an elevated rate in boys, and a third group of studies concluded that boys and girls develop PTSD with equal frequency. Gender differences were also studied by Breslau et al. (1997). Among subjects who had experienced an emotional trauma in their lifetimes, similar percentages of men and women reported that their first incident occurred before age 15 (about 30%). Within this group, a significantly higher percentage of women (27%) reported rape, assault, or repetitive physical or sexual abuse compared with men (8%). On the other hand, men reported a higher percentage of childhood exposure to serious accidents or injuries. However, these experiences did not predispose either gender to PTSD. Along the spectrum of emotional traumas, women endorsed higher rates of PTSD than did men.

The National Women's Study, a prospective, multivariate analysis, studied 3,006 women to identify separate risk factors for rape and physical assault and the factors that predisposed the victim to developing a corresponding PTSD syndrome (Acierno et al. 1999). Past victimization, minority ethnic status, and preexisting PTSD significantly increased a woman's risk of being sexually assaulted. A different set of risk factors were then found to correlate with developing PTSD secondary to the rape, including history of depression, alcohol abuse, or having incurred a physical injury during the assault. A distinct set of risk factors for physical assault, and PTSD secondary to that assault, were also identified.

Pfefferbaum (1997) surveyed various other factors that affect a child's response to a traumatic event, including the characteristics of the stressor and exposure to it; individual factors such as gender, age, developmental level, and psychiatric history; family characteristics; and social factors. The trauma response is affected by the emotional and physical proximity of exposure. Physical proximity refers to the relative distance between the observer or victim and the traumatic event. On the other hand, emotional proximity refers to the personal nature of the trauma. For example, an event affecting a loved one would be more traumatic than one affecting a stranger.

There are reportedly also qualitative differences in how various age groups respond to the same traumatic event, such as a school shooting. Older children are more likely to suffer reexperiencing and hyperarousal symptoms, whereas younger children have a greater predilection for avoidance symptoms. Moreover, younger children tend to develop reexperiencing symptoms spontaneously, whereas older children and adults usually did so in response to specific trauma-related cues (Schwarz and Kowalski 1991).

PTSD in adolescence can be particularly damaging from a developmental perspective. The necessary tasks of developing independence and self-sufficiency can be delayed or permanently impaired. In addition, PTSD places the teenager at increased risk of alcohol or drug abuse, which in turn elevates the risk of exposure to further trauma, legal difficulties, and other adverse events (Deykin 1999).

Studies have demonstrated that the nature of the trauma has a significant impact on the risk of PTSD and the resulting symptoms. Childhood sexual abuse has been extensively studied and has been shown to cause various adverse psychiatric outcomes. The characteristics in a particular victim seem to depend, at least in part, on several variables. The types of sexual abuse that appear to cause the greatest emotional trauma involve the use of physical force, genital contact, or perpetration by a male authority figure such as a father or stepfather. Sexual abuse involving a family member or other loved one is more traumatic than that involving a stranger, all else being equal. Younger children appear to suffer greater psychologic harm (Browne and Finkelhor 1986).

Numerous authors have postulated a strong association between child sexual abuse and subsequent prostitution. The hypothesized link has been reformulated as a failure in social attachments in the family setting, inappropriate parenting, or both. Using a series of logistical models, researchers examined various background factors for predictive value in measuring the likelihood of prostitution: nontraditional family structure, negative home life, sexual abuse, physical abuse, parental substance abuse, and sexual precocity. Only negative home life and sexual precocity were significant predictive factors. The same factors also predicted which adolescents would become runaways. Sexual abuse did not add a qualitatively distinct factor beyond its contribution to negative home life and sexual precocity (Brannigan and Gibbs Van Brunschot 1997).

Foster care constitutes a substantial and understudied reservoir of child trauma cases. There are approximately a half million children in foster care, 83.4% of whom entered the foster care system at an average age of 3 years. The under-5 age group is the fasting growing segment of the foster care population. Primary issues for these children include a history of physical abuse, sexual abuse, neglect, and abandonment (Benoit 2000).

Children in the foster care system are thus presumably at increased risk of developing PTSD. A recent study compared three groups of 50 foster care children each. One group had a history of physical abuse, the second had a history of sexual abuse, and the third group had no history of abuse. The percentages of subjects who met diagnostic criteria for PTSD were 42%, 64%, and 18%, respectively. The elevated rate of PTSD in the nonabused group was presumably due to other types of traumatic experiences, such as a prior history of witnessing domestic violence (Dubner and Motta 1999).

Researchers have also evaluated the psychologic trauma imposed by childhood cancer. Stuber et al. (1997) studied 186 childhood cancer survivors ages 8–20 years. Although most patients developed at least mild PTSD, the most important factors in predicting persistent symptoms were anxiety and subjective appraisals of life threat and treatment intensity. More objective factors, including biologic relapse, bone marrow transplantation, and age at first diagnosis were not significant. The mothers' perceptions had significant impacts on the pediatric patients' own subjective appraisals of their situations. This suggests the importance of active mental health interventions with both the child patient and the mother during the acute treatment phase. In the context of personal injury litigation, the emotional distress of the mother in the case of a severely ill child potentially translates into additional damages with regard to a trickle-down effect on her sick child.

A recent study suggests that the risk of PTSD for a child victim in a motor vehicle accident has been underappreciated and is in fact similar to that encountered in violent crimes (de Vries et al. 1999). Using a prospective cohort study of children and adolescents who were physically injured in traffic accidents, the researchers found that 25% of victims qualified for a diagnosis of PTSD. Of note, the severity of the physical injuries did not correlate with the development of PTSD. Rather, child victims who were in the older age range or whose accompanying parent developed PTSD were at increased risk. The child's reliance on the parent for affect modulation is again seen, as in the cancer study described above.

There is a growing body of literature examining the relationship between subtance use disorders and PTSD in adolescents. For example, Deykin and Buka (1997) studied 297 adolescents in a residential drug treatment program who qualified for a diagnosis of alcohol or drug dependence. The subjects endorsed a 74.4% rate of trauma exposure and a lifetime PTSD prevalence of 29.6%. Among males, the primary disorder appeared to be substance dependence, which presumably led to high-risk behaviors and environmental settings that predisposed them to emotional trauma. In contrast, in the girls, trauma was followed by substance dependence, suggesting that the latter may represent self-medication for PTSD or an example of high-risk behavior in response to trauma. Major depressive disorder was the most common comorbid condition with PTSD.

Preliminary studies suggest that individuals who have reduced cognitive function may be at increased risk for developing PTSD in two ways. First, they may be at increased risk of exposure to a traumatic event, for example, because of decreased judgment. Second, such individuals may be at increased risk of developing PTSD following a given traumatic stimulus compared with the average person. The authors suggested that this effect may be caused by a difference in how the traumatic experience is encoded or in coping skills (Orr and Pitman 1999).

Racial and cultural factors are potentially significant in evaluation and treatment of PTSD but have not been adequately studied. For example, the mental health needs of Latino children and families in the United States are substantially underserved. This population is rapidly increasing because of high birth rates and rapid immigration. Latino youth are at increased risk for mental health disorders, including PTSD, because of the high rates of poverty, gang and other violence, pregnancy, and school delinquency or dropout. Immigrants from Central America are particularly vulnerable, having left war-torn homelands for the United States, where they have limited educational, financial, social, and other resources. The genesis of PTSD may be related to factors in the home country, the immigration process, and after arrival in the United States. Garrison et al. (1999) reviewed studies of the mental health effects of immigration on Latino children. The acculturation process affected women and children more adversely than men. Interestingly, the psychiatric resilience of children, particularly small children and teenagers, depended primarily on the response of the mother to stress.

Psychophysiology

Various psychophysiologic alterations in response to trauma have been reported. Some are stable across age or gender, whereas others are particular to specific subpopulations. Abnormalities have included autonomic hyperactivity, lack of habituation to startle stimuli, reduced response to event-related potentials, multiple neurotransmitter system changes, altered hypothalamic-pituitary-adrenal axis functioning, neuropsychologic deficits in memory functions, decreased immune activity, and neuroanatomic abnormalities on structural and functional imaging. Several findings particular to children have been reported as well, including multiple neuroendocrine changes, alterations in the limbic system, and disturbances on electroencephalogram (Glaser 2000; van der Kolk 1997).

One of the most promising domains of research into the biology of PTSD has involved the measurement of increased physiologic responsiveness to trauma-related cues, exploiting DSM-IV Criterion B(5). Roughly two-thirds of patients with a DSM-IV diagnosis of PTSD demonstrate this heightened reactivity.

The situation is complex. Individuals with specific phobia or a past history of PTSD that is now asymptomatic may experience the same physiologic reactivity to trauma-related cues as a patient who currently meets PTSD criteria. It is possible to retain this reactivity but no longer meet the criteria for PTSD. This implies that a patient's responsiveness to treatment should not be based on whether he or she experiences a resolution of this heightened reactivity. Arguably, the same could be said for a jury reward of monetary damages in a civil case involving a history of now asymptomatic PTSD that meets criterion B(5) by laboratory indices.

Physiologic reactivity is also affected by symptom severity in current PTSD. Individuals with mild disorders collectively have a decreased prevalence of physiologic reactivity in response to trauma-related cues, reducing the sensitivity of such measures in the PTSD population as a whole. On the other hand, patients with moderate to severe PTSD almost uniformly demonstrate this phenomenon (Orr 1997).

A related area is the study of neurophysiologic markers of sexual abuse and other childhood traumas in adult survivors. Physiologic reactivity of women with a history of childhood sexual abuse was investigated by Metzger et al. (1999) using heart rate, skin conductance, and EMG responses to startling tones. Three groups were compared: those with current PTSD, those with a lifetime history of PTSD but no current symptoms, and those with no history of PTSD. Reactivity, as measured by elevated heart rate, greater skin conductance magnitudes, and slower absolute habituation of skin conductance responses, was found to be abnormal in both the current PTSD and lifetime PTSD groups but not in the no-PTSD group. The findings were consistent after controlling for medication use and anxiety and depressive symptoms, suggesting that physiologic reactivity may represent a core feature of PTSD. The fact that the same abnormalities persisted after the PTSD symptoms remitted (in the lifetime PTSD group) indicates that the reactivity may either represent a predisposition to PTSD or a fixed derangement that persists as a by-product of PTSD (Metzger et al. 1999). Given the present state of research, biologic markers of physiologic reactivity to trauma-related cues are not a reliable diagnostic tool in children or adolescents (American Academy of Child and Adolescent Psychiatry 1998).

Assessment

General guidelines for the clinical assessment of PTSD in children and adolescents are available and provide part of the foundation for forensic examination (American Academy of Child and Adolescent Psychiatry 1998; Newman et al. 1996; Perrin et al. 2000). A wide variety of assessment instruments are available to assist the evaluator in the diagnosis of PTSD, including structured clinical interviews, clinician-administered scales, patient self-report checklists, and personality inventories such as the Minnesota Multiphasic Personality Inventory–2 and its PTSD subscales (Newman et al. 1996). The American Academy of Child and Adolescent Psychiatry (AACAP) has adopted assessment standards for evaluating PTSD in children and adolescents. Although there are a large number of teacher, parent, and patient self-report scales and other tools available, these adjunctive instruments are imperfect and should not serve as a substitute for a detailed interview by an experienced clinician (American Academy of Child and Adolescent Psychiatry 1998).

The AACAP notes that one of the most confounding issues is the variable symptom expression in younger age groups. The number and proportion of reexperiencing, avoidance and numbing, and hyperarousal symptoms can vary considerably, such that a child may have dramatic symptoms in one category and seem to have few or no symptoms in another category. The research remains unclear whether a so-called partial PTSD syndrome is functionally any different from a cluster of symptoms that meets full DSM-IV diagnostic criteria.

The evaluation of a child or adolescent for PTSD in a medical-legal setting is fraught with dangers and potential pitfalls. Issues include bias (whether intentional or not), qualifications to perform such an evaluation, and the manner in which the evaluation is conducted and the results are transmitted.

In general, the roles of treating clinician and forensic expert dare not mix (Strasburger et al. 1997). The psychiatrist who provides patient care serves as the patient's advocate, accepts the child's reports at face value, and concentrates on perceptions rather than facts. The medical-legal expert, on the other hand, in theory should be unbiased, more objective in his or her quest, and have the education, training, and experience to address such factors as exaggeration, secondary gain, and corroboration through testing, third-party interviews, and review of records. Although guidelines have been suggested for clinical evaluation of PTSD in minors (American Academy of Child and Adolescent Psychiatry 1998), the experienced forensic expert must adapt and extend these parameters to meet the medical-legal context at hand.

Quinn (1995) addressed the issue of forensic examination of the child or adolescent. She examined various features unique to PTSD in children, the forensic assessment process, and the importance of adequate qualifications to perform such a specialized evaluation, particularly in prepubertal children. She stressed the importance of a developmental perspective in properly eliciting and understanding the child's signs and symptoms of PTSD. Indeed, Pynoos et al. (1996) noted that "the critical link between traumatic stress and personality is the formation of trauma-related expectations as these are expressed in the thoughts, emotions, behaviors, and biology of the developing child" (p. 332).

Quinn (1995) pointed out that in a forensic assessment, several factors may lead to the under- and overreporting of emotional trauma, and hence PTSD, in children. Factors that artificially lower the rate of detection include denial or minimization by parents, teachers, and other adults; frequent lack of reporting by children; and ignorance in adults about the frequency and presentations of child PTSD. An inability to appreciate or elicit clues to PTSD in younger children with limited verbal expressiveness will also hamper the detection process.

Other factors may inappropriately elevate the frequency with which childhood emotional trauma is reported. These include low thresholds for mandatory reporting; biases and inadequate training in trauma-oriented therapists; and incompetent, biased, or inadequate clinical and forensic examinations.

PTSD and Memory

Memory is affected by two PTSD-related disorders. First, the individual is primed to receive intrusive, repetitive, and unwanted reexperiencing symptoms through flashbacks, memories, nightmares, and similar phenomena. Second, patients may experience psychogenic amnesia in which significant information about the traumatic event is inaccessible to the individual despite an otherwise intact memory apparatus (McNally 1997). In McNally's (1997) study, recall of traumatic memory was assessed in adult survivors of childhood sexual abuse using a directed forgetting paradigm. Individuals demonstrated intact recall of trauma-related information, whereas persistent rumination about the trauma that affects concentration may impair the ability to encode and recall nontraumatic material.

In her review of the literature on childhood trauma and memory from the perspective of a child forensic psychiatrist, Quinn (1995) pointed to a number of memory disturbances seen in this population. These disturbances consisted of five different entities: 1) omitting moments of most severe life threat; 2) distorting the chronology and characteristics of the trauma event; 3) the presence of omens or premonitions; 4) denial, minimization, or suppression of experiences; and 5) dissociative memory disturbances.

The neural correlates of pathologic memories of childhood sexual abuse have also been studied in women with and without PTSD. In one such study, subjects were exposed to neutral and trauma-related cues while undergoing positron emission tomography. When compared with women without PTSD, the women who qualifed for a diagnosis of PTSD demonstrated dysfunction in multiple areas of the brain, including the medial prefrontal cortex, hippocampus, and visual association cortex (Bremner et al. 1999).

Ash and Derdeyn (1997) reviewed the literature on suggestibility and the veracity of child victim testimony in sexual abuse cases. They concluded that "results generally support the finding that children are able to recall well, but that younger children, especially preschool children, are more susceptible to suggestion and misleading questions than older children or adults" (p. 1496). They noted that the context of the evaluation is important in assessing validity of a child victim's claims: "There is an increasing awareness that allegations (of child sexual abuse) may be false, especially when the allegation arises in the context of a contested custody or visitation dispute or arises after multiple 'sexual abuse evaluation' interviews of groups of suspected victims" (p. 1496).

The available research data, and public opinion, on the reliability of recovered adult memories of childhood physical and sexual abuse as well as child witness testimony of victimization remain heated and controversial. These topics have been reviewed in detail by G.S. Goodman et al. (1999). They explained that, according to the reconstructionist perspective, there are three components to memory: acquisition, retention, and retrieval. *Acquisition* refers to the assimilation or encoding of information into memory. *Retention* pertains to storage of that information. *Retrieval* involves the ability to access that stored information at a later time. Memory difficulties that adversely affect the reliability of a child or adult witness's testimony or subjective self-reports in psychotherapy can occur at any or all three stages.

With regard to acquisition of data to be stored in memory, the complexity and emotional valence of an event, such as a violent crime, can disturb the ability to adequately pay attention to and to encode all relevant information. Key information will be stored at the expense of ancillary details first. Other factors can obviously affect attentiveness as well, including head injury, prescription medications, intoxication with illicit substances, or an underlying medical condition. Retention of stored information can fall prey to a variety of perturbations. Two key factors are forgetting and postevent contamination with additional, inaccurate information. The risk of forgetting increases with the passage of time, appears to be more of a problem in younger children, and is greater when the information is impersonal or peripheral as opposed to highly personal, relevant experiences. The insinuation of inaccurate postevent data into the victim's memory can occur through various means, including overhearing police officers, parents, or other adults discussing the event; listening to or reading police or legal reports; obtaining information from the news media; and being subjected to leading but inaccurate interviews (G.S. Goodman et al. 1999).

A primary concern with regard to retrieval of information is suggestibility. Children are in general more susceptible to this process, particularly in a high-stress situation such as the courtroom or in front of a high-status interviewer. The manner in which a forensic examiner or attorney questions a child may have a significant impact through intimidation, misleading questions with false premises, or overly adult formulations and vocabulary (G.S. Goodman et al. 1999). Indeed, the process of testifying as a trauma victim in civil litigation or a criminal trial can be highly stressful, even traumatic, for the child (Eth 1988).

Despite the wealth of ways in which patient or witness testimony can be distorted, the issue of recovered or repressed memories remained unsolved. There are adults who can indeed repress and then later uncover genuine memories of childhood traumas, just as there are individuals who can supposedly retrieve recollections of childhood abuse, often through inappropriate therapist prompting, that have no basis in fact (G.S. Goodman et al. 1999). Although the matter may never admit to a single solution, careful outside corroboration of these memories is the cornerstone of proper evaluation.

Contrary to general opinion, the fact that a victim has a prior history of major mental illness, such as bipolar disorder or schizophrenia, does not per se invalidate or reduce the veracity of the victim's report of a violent crime (L.A. Goodman et al. 1999). L.A. Goodman et al. (1999) studied victims of childhood sexual abuse as well as adult rape and physical assault who had histories of active major mental illnesses. Overall, when careful examination techniques were used, a reliable account of the traumatic experience or its emotional sequelae was obtainable in most cases.

Treatment

Pfefferbaum (1997) recommended that consideration be given to treatment for PTSD even when only partial diagnostic criteria are met. The full symptom complex may not develop until later. Furthermore, PTSD syndromes in children can have a chronic course that adversely affects important developmental strides. Thus, just as the child plaintiff who fails to meet adequate DSM-IV criteria for PTSD may still be entitled to comparable emotional damages because of the event itself, he or she may also be rewarded a more aggressive future treatment package based on such authoritative articles that blur the distinction between partial and full PTSD syndromes.

A variety of treatment modalities are available for PTSD, including psychosocial interventions, cognitive-behavioral psychotherapy, in vivo and imaginal exposure techniques, eye movement desensitization and reprocessing, and pharmacotherapy. Drug therapy serves to both improve certain core symptoms, such as insomnia, and render patients more amenable to the anxiety-provoking side effects of the psychological treatments. The adult literature on medication management is tentative, based largely on uncontrolled studies. Selective serotonin reuptake inhibitors are considered first-line broad-spectrum agents for PTSD and common comorbidites, whereas benzodiazepines, tricyclic antidepressants, monoamine oxidase inhibitors, and clonidine are some of the more frequently used secondary agents (Papp 2000). Unfortunately, pharmacotherapy of PTSD in children and adolescents, particularly prepubertal children, is based on too few reliable studies to generate specific recommendations. General approaches and medication choices are extrapolated from the research data and clinical experience on adults with PTSD (Donnelly et al. 1999).

Conclusions and Recommendations

PTSD, the signature of emotional trauma for many victims, is a potent force in criminal and civil proceedings and yet remains poorly understood and inadequately defined in many ways in children and adolescents. The advent of PTSD as a psychiatric diagnosis revolutionized emotional personal injury claims for the plaintiff's attorney (Stone 1993). What had seemed to be largely intangible, subjective, and vague now had the legitimacy of biology and medicine. In the jury's eyes, PTSD is now a genuine medical disorder, akin to heart attack or hip fracture. It furthermore solved the issue of causation because it is incident specific—the plaintiff developed intrusive memories, nightmares, and other symptoms referable to the traumatic event in question. Yet expert examination and testimony about PTSD in the young is a potentially perilous undertaking to the biased, overzealous, or underqualified psychiatrist.

Proper forensic evaluation of children and adolescents requires that certain general and context-specific principles be followed when making or ruling out a diagnosis of PTSD. The expert must do his or her best to preserve neutrality and objectivity and to stay within the confines of the psychiatrist's role and expertise. Because the psychiatrist does not sit in the courtroom as trier of fact, he or she must avoid temptations in both reports and testimony to opine about ultimate issues that involve legal conclusions.

For example, the expert can provide valuable information as to whether the subject has the mental *capacity* from a psychiatric standpoint to make a certain type of decision or perform a particular task. Whether the subject in question ultimately has the *competency* to do so is the purview of the judge or jury. In other words, the expert gives testimony that is *relevant* to whether a particular legal test or criterion is met and that is within his or her education, training, and experience. The application of that test or criterion resides with the factfinder.

Likewise, the expert must appreciate that he or she is not there to give the facts of what happened based on what is pieced together in the psychiatric examination. The court only seeks information from the medical-psychiatric body of knowledge that may be helpful to the judge's or jury's decision-making process. Whether the child subject was actually sexually abused at the aunt's house 2 years earlier is beyond the scope of psychiatric opinion and testimony.

However, with that in mind, it is important for forensic examiners to also appreciate the pressures on them, whether subtle or overt, to serve as quasi-investigators for the attorney or law enforcement agency. A criminal or civil case referral may contain an alternative, hidden agenda of data gathering to use against the civil or criminal defendant with no legitimate mental health purpose. Despite all the caveats given above regarding the limits of expert testimony, psychiatrists should be aware that their testimony may have far-reaching implications. For example, information about the emotional sequelae of alleged sexual abuse in a civil trial may trigger a criminal prosecution that previously had been stalled or unplanned (Melton et al. 1997).

Based on the child and adolescent PTSD literature surveyed herein, several more specific cautions and recommendations can be made on behalf of the expert psychiatrist who serves in a forensic consulting capacity. Before the consultation process begins, several issues must be addressed. One is to clarify with the referral source the nature and extent of the consultation and what particular questions are to be addressed. Hidden agendas and police roles are to be avoided. Another pertains to the psychiatrist's qualifications. Depending on the specifics of the case, potential experts must honestly evaluate their own education, training, and experience within child or adolescent psychiatry and then with regard to the particular issues of the case. As Quinn (1995) noted, children, particularly prepubertal children, are not little adults, and adequate qualifications in the field are required. More specialized expertise may also be a prerequisite, beginning with child psychiatry, narrowing to PTSD, and then narrowing further to a certain specialty within PTSD, such as PTSD secondary to child sexual abuse.

Once a civil or criminal consultation referral is accepted, the most basic downfall would be to uncritically equate PTSD with a stereotypic traumatic event followed by the classic triad of reexperiencing, avoidance and numbing, and hyperarousal symptoms. This perspective reflects neither the complex and variable phenomenology of child and adolescent PTSD nor the relative strengths and weaknesses of the research support for various domains of traumatic experience and resultant psychopathology. The expert must, for example, have an appreciation for the different faces of PTSD. The child may not meet all three prongs of the triad of PTSD symptoms at a particular time, and the relative proportions of symptoms may fluctuate substantially over time. The presentation of the disorder may be delayed, or it may come and go. Some DSM-IV symptoms may not apply, and other expressions of the trauma experience, such as generalized nightmares or nonspecific fears of the dark, may predominate. As the AACAP (1998) noted, a partial PTSD syndrome may functionally, and thus for the purposes of civil damages, be the essentially the same as the full disorder. The risk of developing PTSD depends in part on the trauma and other factors and can fluctuate considerably. Variability is the rule; a textbook presentation may be the exception.

There must also be an appreciation for the outside factors that affect the child PTSD victim, distinct from the typical adult case. As discussed above, several qualitatively different types of studies demonstrated the central importance of the parent's emotional reaction to the trauma in modulating the outcome for the child.

Whether the trauma is cancer or a car accident, the child will, to a degree, look to mother for comfort and a coping model. A greater posttraumatic emotional reaction in the parent will have potentially negative consequences for the child's symptomatology, response to treatment, and long-term prognosis.

The expert must also accept the limits of the scientific literature in child and adolescent PTSD. For example, many of the studies in adults pertaining to psychopharmacology, memory, and neurophysiology of PTSD are not necessarily applicable to children and teenagers, particularly younger children. There is a paucity of controlled studies for various cultures and ethnic minorities, limiting the scientific foundation for much testimony in these populations.

Finally, the potential pitfalls in child victim testimony have been reviewed. Although the child or adolescent witness has many strengths, there are a number of avenues by which his or her memory of events can be truncated or contaminated. The legal system unfortunately fosters such problems by allowing intimidation, inappropriate cross-examination, and other adversities. The final trauma may lie in the adjudication of the PTSD itself.

References

Acierno R, Resnick H, Kilpatrick DG, et al: Risk factors for rape, physical assault, and posttraumatic stress disorder in women: examination of differential multivariate relationships. J Anxiety Disord 13:541–563, 1999

American Academy of Child and Adolescent Psychiatry: Practice parameters for the assessment and treatment of children and adolescents with posttraumatic stress disorder. J Am Acad Child Adolesc Psychiatry 37(suppl): 4S–26S, 1998

American Psychiatric Association: Diagnostic and Statistical Manual of Mental Disorders. Washington, DC, American Psychiatric Association, 1952

American Psychiatric Association: Diagnostic and Statistical Manual of Mental Disorders, 2nd Edition. Washington, DC, American Psychiatric Association, 1968

American Psychiatric Association: Diagnostic and Statistical Manual of Mental Disorders, 3rd Edition. Washington, DC, American Psychiatric Association, 1980

American Psychiatric Association: Diagnostic and Statistical Manual of Mental Disorders, 3rd Edition Revised. Washington, DC, American Psychiatric Association, 1987

American Psychiatric Association: Diagnostic and Statistical Manual of Mental Disorders, 4th Edition. Washington, DC, American Psychiatric Association, 1994

American Psychiatric Association: Diagnostic and Statistical Manual of Mental Disorders, 4th Edition, Text Revision. Washington, DC, American Psychiatric Association, 2000

Ash P, Derdeyn AP: Forensic child and adolescent psychiatry: a review of the past 10 years. J Am Acad Child Adolesc Psychiatry 36:1493–1502, 1997

Benoit MB: Foster care, in Kaplan and Sadock's Comprehensive Textbook of Psychiatry. Edited by Sadock BJ, Sadock VA. Philadelphia, PA, Lippincott Williams and Wilkins, 2000, pp 2873–2877

Blank AS: The longitudinal course of posttraumatic stress disorder, in Posttraumatic Stress Disorder: DSM-IV and Beyond. Edited by Davidson JRT, Foa EB. Washington, DC, American Psychiatric Press, 1993, pp 3–22

Boehnlein JK: The process of research in posttraumatic stress disorder. Perspectives in Biology and Medicine 32:455–465, 1989

Brady KT, Killeen TK, Brewerton T, et al: Comorbidity of psychiatric disorders and posttraumatic stress disorder. J Clin Psychiatry 61(suppl): 22–32, 2000

Brannigan A, Gibbs Van Brunschot E: Youthful prostitution and child sexual trauma. Int J Law Psychiatry 20:337–354, 1997

Bremner JD, Narayan M, Staib LH, et al: Neural correlates of memories of childhood sexual abuse in women with and without posttraumatic stress disorder. Am J Psychiatry 156:1787–1795, 1999

Breslau N, Davis GC, Andreski P, et al: Sex differences in posttraumatic stress disorder. Arch Gen Psychiatry 54:1044–1048, 1997

Brett EA, Spitzer RL, Williams JBW: DSM-III-R criteria for posttraumatic stress disorder. Am J Psychiatry 145:1232–1236, 1988

Browne A, Finkelhor D: Impact of child sexual abuse: a review of the research. Psychol Bull 99:66–77, 1986

de Vries AP, Kassam-Adams N, Cnaan A, et al: Looking beyond the physical injury: posttraumatic stress disorder in children and parents after pediatric traffic injury. Pediatrics 104:1293–1299, 1999

Deykin EY: Posttraumatic stress disorder in childhood and adolescence: a review. Medscape Mental Health (www.medscape.com) 4:1–11, 1999

Deykin EY, Buka SL: Prevalence and risk factors for posttraumatic stress disorder among chemically dependent adolescents. Am J Psychiatry 154:752–757, 1997

Donnelly CL, Amaya-Jackson L, March JS: Psychopharmacology of pediatric posttraumatic stress disorder. J Child Adolesc Psychopharmacol 9:203–220, 1999

Dubner AE, Motta RW: Sexually and physically abused foster care children and posttraumatic stress disorder. J Consult Clin Psychol 67: 367–373, 1999

Eth S: The child victim as witness in sexual abuse proceedings. Psychiatry 51:221–232, 1988

Garrison EG, Roy IS, Azar V: Responding to the mental health needs of Latino children and families through school-based services. Clin Psychol Rev 19:199–219, 1999

Glaser D: Child abuse and neglect and the brain: a review. J Child Psychol Psychiatry 41:97–116, 2000

Goodman GS, Redlich AD, Qin J, et al: Evaluating eyewitness testimony in adults and children, in The Handbook of Forensic Psychology. Edited by Hess AK, Weiner IB. New York, John Wiley and Sons, 1999, pp 218–272

Goodman LA, Thompson KM, Weinfurt K, et al: Reliability of reports of violent victimization and posttraumatic stress disorder among men and women with serious mental illness. J Trauma Stress 12:587–599, 1999

Harvey AG, Bryant RA: The relationship between acute stress disorder and posttraumatic stress disorder: a 2-year prospective evaluation. J Consult Clin Psychol 67:985–988, 1999

Kessler RC, Sonnega A, Bromet E, et al: Epidemiological risk factors for trauma and PTSD, in Risk Factors for Posttraumatic Stress Disorder. Edited by Yehuda R. Washington, DC, American Psychiatric Press, 1999, pp 23–59

McLeer SV, Callaghan M, Henry D, et al: Psychiatric disorders in sexually abused children. J Am Acad Child Adolesc Psychiatry 33:313–319, 1994

McNally RJ: Implicit and explicit memory for trauma-related information in PTSD. Ann N Y Acad Sci 821:219–224, 1997

McNally RJ, Saigh PA: On the distinction between traumatic simple phobia and posttraumatic stress disorder, in Posttraumatic Stress Disorder: DSM-IV and Beyond. Edited by Davidson JRT, Foa EB. Washington, DC, American Psychiatric Press, 1993, pp 207–212

Melton GB, Petrila J, Poythress NG, et al: Psychological Evaluations for the Courts: A Handbook for Mental Health Professionals, 2nd Edition. New York, Guilford, 1997

Metzger LJ, Orr SP, Berry NJ, et al: Physiologic reactivity to startling tones in women with posttraumatic stress disorder. J Abnorm Psychol 108:347–352, 1999

Newman CJ: Disaster at Buffalo Creek. Children of disaster: clinical observations at Buffalo Creek. Am J Psychiatry 133:306–312, 1976

Newman E, Kaloupek DG, Keane TM: Assessment of posttraumatic stress disorder in clinical and research settings, in Traumatic Stress: The Effects of Overwhelming Experience on Mind, Body, and Society. Edited by van der Kolk BA, McFarlane AC, Weisaeth L. New York, Guilford, 1996, pp 242–275

Orr SP: Psychophysiologic reactivity to trauma-related imagery in PTSD: diagnostic and theoretical implications in recent findings. Ann N Y Acad Sci 821:114–124, 1997

Orr SP, Pitman RK: Neurocognitive risk factors for PTSD, in Risk Factors for Posttraumatic Stress Disorder. Edited by Yehuda R. Washington, DC, American Psychiatric Press, 1999, pp 125–141

Papp LA: Anxiety disorders: somatic treatment, in Kaplan and Sadock's Comprehensive Textbook of Psychiatry. Edited by Sadock BJ, Sadock VA. Philadelphia, PA, Lippincott Williams and Wilkins, 2000, pp 1490–1498

Perrin S, Smith P, Yule W: Practitioner review: the assessment and treatment of post-traumatic stress disorder in children and adolescents. J Child Psychol Psychiatry 41:277–289, 2000

Pfefferbaum B: Posttraumatic stress disorder in children: a review of the past 10 years. J Am Acad Child Adolesc Psychiatry 36:1503–1511, 1997

Pynoos RS, Steinberg AM, Goenjian A: Traumatic stress in childhood and adolescence: recent developments and current controversies, in Traumatic Stress: The Effects of Overwhelming Experience on Mind, Body, and Society. Edited by van der Kolk BA, McFarlane AC, Weisaeth L. New York, Guilford, 1996, pp 331–358

Quinn KM: Guidelines for the psychiatric examination of posttraumatic stress disorder in children and adolescents, in Posttraumatic Stress Disorder in Litigation: Guidelines for Forensic Assessment. Edited by Simon RI. Washington, DC, American Psychiatric Press, 1995, pp 85–98

Schwarz ED, Kowalski JM: Malignant memories: PTSD in children and adults after a school shooting. J Am Acad Child Adolesc Psychiatry 30:936–944, 1991

Stone AA: Post-traumatic stress disorder and the law: critical review of the new frontier. Bulletin of the American Academy of Psychiatry and the Law 21:23–36, 1993

Strasburger LH, Gutheil TG, Brodsky A: On wearing two hats: role conflict in serving as both psychotherapist and expert witness. Am J Psychiatry 154:448–456, 1997

Stuber ML, Kazak AE, Meeske K, et al: Predictors of posttraumatic stress symptoms in childhood cancer survivors. Pediatrics 100:958–964, 1997

Terr LC: Childhood traumas: an outline and overview. Am J Psychiatry 148:10–20, 1991

Terr LC: Children of Chowchilla: a study of psychic trauma. Psychoanal Study Child 34:547–623, 1979

True WR, Lyons MJ: Genetic risk factors for PTSD: a twin study, in Risk Factors for Posttraumatic Stress Disorder. Edited by Yehuda R. Washington, DC, American Psychiatric Press, 1999, pp 68–71

van der Kolk BA: The psychobiology of posttraumatic stress disorder. J Clin Psychiatry 58(suppl):16–24, 1997

Weinstein D, Staffelbach D, Biaggio M: Attention-deficit hyperactivity disorder and posttraumatic stress disorder: differential diagnosis in childhood sexual abuse. Clin Psychol Rev 20:359–378, 2000

Chapter 3

PTSD in Children and Adolescents in the Juvenile Justice System

William Arroyo, M.D.

Introduction

The widespread mental health needs of children and youth in the juvenile justice system has been repeatedly documented since the early 1980s (Knitzer 1982; Society for Adolescent Medicine 2000; Timmons-Mitchell et al. 1997). The incarceration of adults with mental disorders (Ditton 1999; Teplin 1990) is an unfortunate trend that mental health practitioners, policymakers, and advocates fear may also be occurring in the juvenile justice system. This practice has recently triggered a focused interest by the federal government (Cocozza and Skowyra 2000), demonstrated by a series of investigations conducted by the Civil Rights Division of the U.S. Department of Justice (Butterfield 1998).

Such investigations have documented extremely adverse conditions and woefully inadequate services, including mental health services, in juvenile correctional facilities in Georgia, Kentucky, Puerto Rico, and the Mariana Islands resulting in legal settlements and consent decrees (Rosenbaum 1999). Another state, Louisiana, is in litigation regarding similar conditions in its facilities. The recent initiation of the first national survey of juvenile justice facilities by the U.S. Department of Health and Human Services' Center for Mental Health Services (1998) is yet more evidence of a heightened awareness by the federal government. Congress has also entered this arena with the introduction of the bill known as the Mental Health Juvenile Justice Act during the 106th session of Congress in 1999. A national forum on the criminal justice system and mental health was recently co-sponsored by the U.S. Department of Justice (2000) and Substance Abuse and Mental Health Services Administration; national experts from the field were convened to address common concerns. The lack of mental health resources and inadequate conditions in detention facilities has also recently been a focus of the press (Romo 2000).

Demographics

The Census of Juveniles in Residential Placement (CJRP) (Snyder and Sickmund 1999) indicated that, in 1997, 368 of every 100,000 juveniles in the United States (aged 10 to the upper age of juvenile court jurisdiction in each state) or approximately 0.4% of youth were in custody. Juveniles are generally considered to be those who have not reached age 18; this age ceiling may vary in some states. Nearly 70% of juveniles in custody are committed (adjudicated and placed), whereas the remainder are detained (generally awaiting adjudication). A 1-day count of juveniles in custody in 1997 was approximately 106,000. Youth charged with delinquency offenses accounted for 93% of the juvenile offender population, whereas status offenses accounted for the other 7%. California, Texas, and Florida together account for 25% of this population with more than 30% of juveniles in custody.

The number of delinquency cases that involved detention between the point at which youth were referred to court and the disposition of the youth steadily increased between 1987 and 1996 from 231,900 to 320,900 nationwide (Snyder and Sickmund 1999). Regardless of offense, males were more likely to be detained than females in 1996; males accounted for 83% of cases involving detention. Offenses directed at people (e.g., manslaughter, assault) and those related to drugs had the greatest likelihood of detention for males, whereas offenses directed at people and public order offenses were more likely for females placed in detention.

Mental Disorders

The prevalence of clinically important mental disorders is estimated to be at least 12% (Friedman et al. 1996) among the general population of children and youth, with approximately half having severe mental disorders; other investigators estimate a range of 14%–20% (Brandenburg et al. 1990; Institute of Medicine 1989). Large-scale epidemiologic studies of the juvenile justice population have yet to be conducted. Several studies, however, suggested that the prevalence of mental disorders among incarcerated youth exceeds that of the general population of children and youth (Atkins et al. 1999; Timmons-Mitchell et al. 1997). One study (Atkins et al. 1999) suggested that the prevalence rates of psychiatric disturbances among incarcerated youth are very similar to those of clinical populations. Seriously delinquent youth, such as juvenile murderers (Myers et al. 1995) and others (Barnum et al. 1989), have been known to have exceedingly high rates of mental disorders.

Conduct disorder rates have varied widely among juvenile justice populations from as low as 10% to as high as 91% (Cocozza and Ingalls 1984; Halikas et al. 1990; Hollander and Turner 1985; McPherson, unpublished data, 1991). Rates for affective disorders, including dysthymia, major depression, and bipolar disorders, range from 32% to 78% (McPherson, unpublished data, 1991; Student and Myhill, unpublished manuscript, 1986). Anxiety disorders also vary from 6% to 41% (Atkins et al. 1999; McPherson, unpublished data, 1991; Student and Myhill, unpublished manuscript, 1986). Attention deficit disorder rates have been reported from 19% to 46% (Halikas et al. 1990; Hollander and Turner 1985; Student and Myhill, unpublished manuscript, 1986). Rates of alcohol and drug abuse range from 25% to 67% (Halikas et al. 1990; James 1999; Student and Myhill unpublished manuscript, 1986). High prevalence rates for learning disabilities and specific developmental disorders are also noted to range widely from 17% to 53% (Barnum et al. 1989; Hollander and Turner 1985; Robbins et al. 1983; Smykla and Willis 1981).

Comorbidity, including psychotic disturbances and neurocognitive impairment, is apparently also very elevated among the juvenile justice population (Atkins et al. 1999; Barnum et al. 1989; James 1999; Otto et al. 1992). This is not unexpected, given the numerous risk factors such as high poverty rates, physical/sexual assault, neglect, and other significant family factors found among many of these youth (James 1999).

Posttraumatic Stress Disorder

Rates of posttraumatic stress disorder (PTSD) (American Psychiatric Association 1994) among children and youth have been primarily restricted to groups of children who have been exposed to maltreatment (Herman 1992; Kiser et al. 1988), war zones (Arroyo and Eth 1985; Dyregrov et al. 2000; Garbarino and Kostelny 1996), natural disasters (Galante and Foa 1986; Garrison et al. 1993), community disasters (Breton et al. 1993), and single traumatic events (Pynoos et al. 1987; Terr 1989) either as victims or bystanders. Community studies assessing prevalence of PTSD have been almost exclusively conducted on adult populations. A recent study (Giaconia et al. 1995), however, examined the lifetime prevalence of trauma exposure and PTSD among older youth. This study concluded that among the 384 nearly 18-year-old youth, 6.3% met lifetime criteria for PTSD using DSM-III-R (American Psychiatric Association 1987) criteria. This rate falls in the upper range of rates found in community studies on adults, which vary from 1.0% to 1.3% in the Epidemiologic Catchment Area program (Davidson et al. 1991; Helzer et al. 1987) to just over 9.0% in adults ages 21–30 years (Breslau et al. 1991). In addition, the youth study (Giaconia et al. 1995) revealed that those with a lifetime diagnosis of PTSD were at greatest risk for developing problems in several domains as compared with youth exposed to trauma without PTSD and those not exposed at all: "They displayed clinical levels of both internalizing and externalizing behavior problems, performed more poorly academically, reported alarming rates of suicidal ideation and attempts, and had more interpersonal problems and more somatic complaints" (Giaconia et al. 1995, p. 1377). Those who were exposed to traumatic events but did not meet criteria for PTSD nevertheless demonstrated poor functioning in various domains; however, this was to a lesser degree than those with full PTSD. This sample was composed of 99% Euro-Americans from a nonurban working and lower middle class community.

Incarcerated Youth

Studies of PTSD in incarcerated children and youth are rare despite the impressions of several authors (Atkins et al. 1999; Barnum et al. 1989) that this group of children has been exposed to many severe stressors. Four studies (Burton et al. 1994; Cauffman et al. 1998; James 1999; Steiner et al. 1997) on PTSD in incarcerated youth have recently been reported. (These four studies are referred to as "the four studies" throughout the remainder of this chapter.) Two (Cauffman et al. 1998; Steiner et al. 1997) of these studies are of detainees of the California Youth Authority (CYA), which is a secure detention system operated by the State of California primarily for youth who have been adjudicated for very serious crimes; the length of stay in this facility usually exceeds 1 year. These youth have generally been previously arrested and detained at least a few times, and their respective county juvenile courts have determined that they are no longer suitable for county detention facilities, which tend to provide average stays of 4 to 6 months. Juveniles who are tried as adults often spend the remainder of their detention in CYA until they reach their 25th birthday. The other two studies (Burton et al. 1994; James 1999) focus on offenders from secure California county detention facilities, which tend to serve youth offenders who commit less serious crimes than detainees in CYA. Most of the subjects of these four studies were from urban areas. Family members were not interviewed as part of any of the four studies.

The rates for PTSD among incarcerated youth from the four studies ranged from a low of 24% (Burton et al. 1994) to a high of 48.9% (Cauffman et al. 1998). These rates were approximately four to eight times as high as those found in a community sample (Giaconia et al. 1995) (see Table 3–1). Rates of partial PTSD (i.e., patients who meet only some of the diagnostic criteria) were 11.7% (Cauffman et al. 1998) and 20% (Steiner et al. 1997) in two of the four studies; partial PTSD rates were not reported in the other two studies.

Table 3–1. Four studies on PTSD in incarcerated youth

Variables	James 1999	Cauffman et al. 1998	Steiner et al. 1997	Burton et al. 1994
n	200	96	85	74
PTSD, %	28/52[1]	48.9	31.7	24
Partial PTSD, %	Not reported	11.7	20	Not reported
Criteria	LASC[2]	PDI[4]	PDI[4]	DSM-III-R[3]
Age, y	12–20	13–22	13–20	13–18
Median age, y	16[5]	17.2	16.6	16
Gender, m/f	100/100	All females	All males	All males
White, non-Hispanic, %	0	23.3	30.1	10
Hispanic, %	52	28.9	26.9	40
African–American, %	48	21.1	37.6	40
Asian, %	0	4.4	0	7
Other[6], %	0	12.2	5.4	0

[1]Males 28, females 52
[2]Los Angeles Symptom Checklist (Foy et al. 1997)
[3]Diagnostic and Statistical Manual of Mental Disorders, 3rd Edition Revised (American Psychiatric Association 1987)
[4]Psychiatric Diagnostic Interview–Revised, PTSD module
[5]"just below 16"
[6]Biracial or other ethnic/racial group

One study (Steiner et al. 1997) indicated that although many youth of the sample had been referred for a mental health evaluation, none had been referred for symptoms of PTSD; the other three studies did not include referral data.

Female Population

The juvenile justice population is overwhelmingly male (Snyder and Sickmund 1999), which in part explains the paucity of studies of the female youth population. The prevalence of psychologic trauma among females has generally been higher than that among males in community sample studies (Breslau et al. 1991; Dembo et al. 1993); 12.3% was the rate found among a national population of adult women (Resnick et al. 1993). Females in a youth community sample (Giaconia et al. 1995) were found to be six times more likely than males to develop lifetime PTSD even though they were exposed to potentially traumatic events with equal frequency. An alarmingly high PTSD rate of 67% was found in a group of urban adolescent girls (Horowitz et al. 1995).

Two (Cauffman et al. 1998; James 1999) of the four studies discussed earlier included female subjects. These subjects had PTSD rates of approximately 50%, ranging from one and a half (Steiner et al. 1997) to two times the rates of their male counterparts (Burton et al. 1994; James 1999) (see Table 3–1). Only 12% of female subjects in one study (Cauffman et al. 1998) did not report exposure to any traumatic events.

Predisposing Factors

Many of the subjects in the four studies had been exposed to myriad potentially traumatic events, of which one or more may have accounted for the onset of PTSD. These included physical and sexual assaults resulting in injuries, witness to homicide, and other acts of violence. Twenty percent of the female subjects in one of the studies (James 1999) reported having been coerced or forced to have intercourse before the age of 14. A few of the incarcerated subjects identified their own violent acts as the etiology of their PTSD symptoms. In one study of incarcerated youth

(James 1999), 72% reported having been wounded by gunshot or having been the target of a shooting; the comparison of a nonincarcerated urban sample reported a prevalence of 27%. Despite the high exposure rate to potentially traumatic events, many incarcerated subjects did not develop PTSD. Other investigators (Pynoos and Nader 1993) discuss this near-miss phenomenon.

The age at which the subjects in the four studies were exposed to trauma is not described, thereby making it difficult to sort out the developmental impact of each exposure, the subjects' responses, and the possible influences of the trauma on future development. Trauma and the response to that trauma can disrupt a child's development (Schwarz and Kowalski 1991), eventual adaptation, and personality (Nader et al. 1990; Perry 1994).

The prevalence of exposure to community violence is relatively high in urban areas as compared with nonurban areas. One group of investigators (Horowitz et al. 1995) referred to the phenomenon of repeated exposure as "compounded community trauma, " whereas another group referred to it as "chronic, environmentally pervasive violence." Children with repeated or long-standing exposure display Type II trauma reactions (Terr 1991) characterized by massive denial, psychic numbing, self-hypnosis, dissociation, aggression toward the self, identification with the aggressor, and personality changes. Risk factors associated with the development of trauma-related psychopathology (Foy et al. 1996), such as poverty, abuse, neglect, sexual molestation, and witnessing violence, were common among the subjects of the four incarcerated groups.

Varying rates of traumatic exposure have been reported. Forty percent of sixth, eighth, and tenth graders in a large sample (Schwab-Stone et al. 1995) of 2,200 urban children reported exposure to a shooting or stabbing in the past year. Of special note in this study was the association of violence exposure and feeling unsafe with a greater willingness to use physical aggression among boys and with depressed and/or anxious mood among girls. Another group of investigators (Richters and Martinez 1993) examined exposure to violence for 165 urban children ages 6–10 years. Nineteen percent of the first and second graders were victims of violence, whereas 61% had witnessed the perpetration of violence; the fifth and sixth graders had higher rates of victimization (32%) and exposure (72%). Although the prevalence of PTSD was not the focus of this study (Richters and Martinez 1993), in the groups that reported higher distress a positive correlation was found between symptoms of distress, many of which overlapped with PTSD criteria, and being victimized or witnessing violence. In a study (Fitzpatrick and Boldizar 1993) of violence exposure in urban African-American children, a PTSD prevalence of 27% among children and youth ages 7–18 years was reported despite the alarming rate of subjects (43.4%) who had witnessed a murder or experienced another potentially traumatic event. The influence of socioeconomic factors is unclear. The overwhelming majority of subjects of the four studies of incarcerated youth with PTSD were members of lower socioeconomic families.

The association of drug and alcohol abuse, delinquency, and psychiatric conditions is discussed extensively in the literature (Finklehor and Dziuba-Leatherman 1994; Widom and Ames 1994). This group of risk factors was evident in the subjects of the four studies of incarcerated youth discussed previously. Two of the four studies (Burton et al. 1994; James 1999) investigated the prevalence of substance use among the incarcerated sample and compared it with a similar local population of nonincarcerated youth. "Substance abuse" and "drinking too much" were problems for 34.5% and 37% of the incarcerated group, respectively, whereas the comparison group reported rates of 10.2% and 18.4%, respectively (James 1999). An intergenerational pattern of substance abuse was common among the incarcerated youth with substance abuse problems. Of those using drugs, 60% indicated that they would continue to do so after leaving the detention facility. Burton et al. (1994) reported that 83% of their incarcerated sample had "significant substance abuse problems," a rate substantially higher than that of the previous study.

Birth and early developmental histories may shed light on some of the behaviors of these youth. A recent study (Arseneault et al. 2000) found an association between the number of minor physical anomalies plus the number of minor physical anomalies of the oral area and an increased risk of violent delinquency in adolescence beyond the effects of family adversity. None of the four studies of incarcerated youth considered early developmental histories of perinatal difficulties, physical injuries to the head and face, or other early traumas, which are not uncommon among abused incarcerated youth (Lewis et al. 1979). Such injuries may be contributory to the neuropsychiatric status of these youth.

The racial/ethnic distribution of the subjects (Table 3–1) of the four studies was 40% African-American, 41% Hispanic, and the remainder either Asian or of other background. The contribution of racial/ethnic factors to psychopathology in these groups was not a focus of any of the four studies. None of the studies indicated the distribution of PTSD prevalence by racial/ethnic group. Natural disaster research studies report contradictory results regarding racial differences (Garrison et al. 1993). Some studies (Ahmad and Mohammed 1996; DiNicola 1996) have suggested cultural factors may affect how PTSD is manifested.

Although none of the four studies systematically addressed comorbidity, two (Burton et al. 1994; James 1999) addressed substance abuse prevalence as described earlier and one (James 1999) addressed depressive symptoms. Physical punishment, sexual abuse, and low family support were significantly correlated with depression among the total sample. Dating violence was also significantly correlated with depressive symptoms in the female sample of the same (i.e., James 1999).

Supportive family relationships have often served as a protective mechanism for children exposed to trauma (Pynoos and Nader 1989). Two of the four studies (Burton et al. 1994; James 1999) of the incarcerated youth examined the contribution of family factors to the subjects' psychopathology. One study (Burton et al. 1994) found that exposure to both violence and family dysfunction was significantly associated with PTSD symptoms. The other study (James 1999) indicated that the families of the subjects were often characterized by the presence of risk behaviors for criminal behavior combined with the absence of protective factors against delinquency; according to the subjects, their parents and guardians were frequently unaware of the subjects' activities outside the home and failed to provide sufficient structure and appropriate consequences for misbehavior. A 16-year-old female gang member whose father had a lengthy history of criminal behavior had, as a young adolescent, witnessed the homicide of her father and had subsequently developed PTSD. She was identified as a repeat offender in the delinquency court and had a psychiatric history of impulsive aggression and possible bipolar disorder.

None of the four studies on incarcerated youth detail the reactions of parents, particularly with regard to posttraumatic stress. An association between parental symptomatology and that of a child has been noted in other studies (Breton et al. 1993).

Suicidal ideation is not uncommon among incarcerated youth. One study (James 1999) reported a prevalence of suicidal ideation of 10% among the sample, whereas the Latina female contingent reported a rate of 45% at the time of the interview. A suicidal 15-year-old girl who had been placed in a detention facility for a status offense impulsively ingested a cleaning fluid within 12 hours of entering the juvenile hall and was taken to a local public hospital. She convinced the probation officer monitoring her to allow her to use the restroom, and she then jumped from the third-story bathroom window. She survived but sustained several fractures.

Gang membership was a prominent characteristic of two of the four studies' subjects (Burton et al. 1994; James 1999). Reasons for membership given by females were "protection," "other family member participation," and "boyfriend search." Gang participation has implications for multipronged community-based interventions (Thomas et al. in press). Illegal activities such as gun use/involvement were often initiated in junior high school (late middle school) years. Although females in one study (James 1999) were more likely to carry weapons other than guns, they differed from males in that the gun involvement was more strongly associated with the absence of protective factors and high levels of personal physical punishment. The risk for intergenerational complications was evident in a portion of the subjects of the four studies. In one study (James 1999), 15% of the incarcerated youth were parents. The caretaking of the subjects' own children and their parenting skills and knowledge were not systematically addressed in this study.

Interventions

Broad-based interventions are required for children and youth with PTSD in the juvenile justice system. Furthermore, the frequent prevalence of comorbidity among this population suggests that two or more diagnoses must be treated simultaneously. These interventions are classified into three categories: 1) individual, 2) family, and 3) community system for purposes of discussion. Each of these categories overlaps with the others and should be provided concurrently. A discussion of a forensic psychiatric evaluation, which may be necessary for many youths in the juvenile justice system, is beyond the scope of this chapter.

Individual

Multimodal interventions including individual, family, and group therapy as well as psychopharmacology have been used to treat PTSD; a combination is often recommended. Research on the effectiveness of these interventions is extremely limited (Pfefferbaum 1997). No research has been conducted on comorbid PTSD and other mental disorders. Youth who are exposed to a traumatic event may be at risk for developing a broad range of mental disorders (Arroyo and Eth 1996) including brief psychotic disorder, dissociative amnesia, and major depressive disorders, among others.

Youth who enter the juvenile justice system should have regular and standardized clinical assessments (American Academy of Child and Adolescent Psychiatry 1998) systematically addressing traumatic violence, substance use, grief and loss, and family factors, among other areas (James 1999; U.S. Department of Justice 2000). Symptoms of PTSD must be diligently addressed (Steiner et al. 1997) because many youth are afraid of disclosing such information. A recently developed mental health screening instrument, the Massachusetts Youth Screening Instrument–2nd Revision (Grisso and Barnum 2000), is being used in a few detention centers; it includes a scale for traumatic experiences. Corroborative historical information provided by parents is rare in the case of detained youth, especially in the clinical realm. This information should be routinely solicited.

A great deal of the literature on treatment focuses on the management of PTSD related to a single traumatic event (Goenjian et al. 1995; Pynoos and Eth 1986) and which treatment ideally should be provided soon after exposure to the event. Certain aspects of these interventions may be applicable, especially in instances in which a recent single exposure has occurred. Direct exploration of the event(s) is always recommended in the context of a safe and trusting environment. Carefully framed questions have been incorporated into an interview protocol (Stein and Lewis 1992) that more successfully elicits physical abuse data among delinquent youth than does direct inquiry. In many instances a combination of different strategies may be indicated, including psychodynamic therapy, anxiety/stress management techniques, cognitive-behavioral therapy, and play therapy (Pfefferbaum 1997). Repeated exposure to trauma during childhood often complicates the recovery process and may result in personality changes (Terr 1991).

Many community-based clinicians are frequently discouraged by juvenile justice youth who appear to be defiant or resistant and display an annoying veneer of bravado. This posture may be a manifestation of avoidance, a core symptom of PTSD. A well-seasoned clinician will often elicit fears, reexperience phenomena, physiologic hyperarousal, depression, grief, and even guilt that result in significant suffering despite an initial hostile demeanor on the part of the youth. A series of prior traumatic events may contribute to the clinical presentation. Establishing trust will often initiate a therapeutic dialogue with such a youngster.

Ongoing revenge fantasies must be addressed in the context of the youth's reality (i.e., reentry to the delinquency court system). Monitoring of suicidal ideation must be ongoing for traumatized youth, especially females (Cauffman et al. 1998; James 1999). Grief precipitated by a traumatic loss should also be a focus of treatment. Bereavement is often prolonged in such instances. The focus on the traumatic aspects should precede that of the grieving process (Eth and Pynoos 1985; Pynoos and Nader 1993) in treatment.

Cognitive assumptions relevant to the traumatic event(s) should be explored (Berliner 1997; Pynoos and Eth 1986). Faulty assumptions related to, for example, culpability, are very common and should be challenged in treatment. Dissociative symptoms are often difficult to distinguish from psychotic states; hallucinations and disorganized thinking are common symptoms in these latter states. Dissociative symptoms should be viewed in the context of trauma and different treatment options from those typical of a psychotic disorder. Forcible administration of medication and/or physical restraint may further traumatize the youth. Caution must be used in the treatment of these symptoms (Putnam 1997).

Various forms of stress management techniques may be paired with trauma-focused discussions. Stress management techniques include progressive muscle relaxation, positive imagery, deep breathing, and thought-stopping exercises that could be taught prior to very detailed discussions of the events (Deblinger and Heflin 1996).

Many youth who have been repeatedly exposed to trauma may not develop PTSD yet may have great difficulty functioning in at least a few domains (Burton et al. 1994; Giaconia 1995; Steiner et al. 1997). This phenomenon may reflect lessened reactivity relative to first-time exposure (Yehuda and McFarlane 1995) or desensitization phenomena.

An investigation (Steiner et al. 1997) of incarcerated youth with PTSD strongly suggested that youth with PTSD have significant problems with impulse control and aggression, which may in turn have adverse implications for recidivism. This trait of reduced restraint, in combination with inappropriate and high reactivity induced by PTSD, is similar to the notion of reactive violence often found in juveniles. Beliefs shared by youth that support the legitimacy and necessity of violence place them at further risk of reoffending (James 1999). These ideas warrant a detailed discussion in psychotherapy. Some youth may require more intensive monitoring and intervention. Implications for the treatment of these traumatized delinquent youths may entail close collaboration with probation personnel. Community programming rooted in youths' accountability and responsibility has demonstrated great promise in decreasing recidivism (Thomas et al. in press).

A sense of a foreshortened future (James 1999) is not atypical and should also be addressed. Various techniques including relaxation, desensitization, and even forms of play therapy should be considered for this population. Although certain forms of play therapy such as drawing activities tend to be more ideal with children (Terr 1989) as opposed to adolescents, many adolescents can be engaged in therapeutic drawing activities.

Eye movement desensitization and reprocessing (EMDR) has shown some effectiveness among adults, but there are no controlled studies regarding the risks and benefits of EMDR in children and adolescents.

Substance abuse services must address the extremely high prevalence of both marijuana and alcohol abuse in this population (James 1999) as well as the use of other illicit substances. These interventions should be provided simultaneously with treatment for the co-occurring mental disorders.

Reevaluation to determine progress and for further follow-up must be included before discharge from custody. Case management may be a key service for youth and families who have several service needs.

Group

Group treatment techniques (Eth et al. 1993; Galante and Foa 1986) may be appropriate for the juvenile justice population when several youth are exposed to a common traumatic event such as the suicide of a detainee in an institution. Group work is very useful for providing information about symptoms, for generating age-appropriate discussions about the course of posttraumatic stress, and for sharing of experiences. Coping strategies can also be shared. The setting of clear limits for the expression of anger and aggression may also be indicated. These techniques may also be useful for triaging those who require more extensive assessment and treatment. Traumatized custodial staff at detention facilities for youth may also benefit from this technique.

Pharmacotherapy

Pharmacotherapy is rarely the sole type of intervention for youth with PTSD (Arroyo and Eth 1996). It serves as an adjunctive form of treatment providing symptomatic relief. Sertraline (Brady et al. 2000), however, has been conclusively shown to be safe and effective in adults and is the only medication that has U.S. Food and Drug Administration approval for the treatment of PTSD in adults. Many classes of medications have been shown to relieve some of the symptoms of PTSD.

The conclusions of studies on the general use of benzodiazepines in children are limited because of high placebo rates, small sample sizes, and very brief medication trials (Riddle et al. 1999). Behavioral disinhibition and paradoxical reactions (Kutcher et al. 1992) are not uncommon, and thus prescribing such medications to youth who often have difficulty with impulse control may be contraindicated. Some authors suggest that benzodiazepines (Lucas and Pasley 1969) may be useful, yet caution is advised (Allen et al. 1993).

Studies involving tricyclic and monoamine oxidase inhibitor antidepressants (Davidson et al. 1990; Frank et al. 1988) suggest some efficacy in adults, especially in regard to the positive symptoms of reexperience phenomena and hyperarousal symptoms. Adrenergic blockers (Kinzie and Leung 1989) such as propranolol and clonidine (Kolb et al. 1984) may also be effective for these symptoms in adults. Clonazepam (Biederman 1987) has been described in case reports as being useful for panic disorder in children and therefore might be another cautious option. Other psychotropic drugs may be indicated for the treatment of comorbid conditions. Combination of psychotropics for use in children and adolescents is a poorly investigated field. Judicious use and close monitoring are strongly recommended. Informed consent and authority for treatment with psychotropic agents vary among jurisdictions; these may rest with parents, delinquency court judges, or sometimes both.

Attitudes toward the use of psychotropic agents by adolescents may influence compliance with medication. Nearly 50% of a large sample (Williams et al. 1998) of incarcerated female adolescents were skeptical about the benefits of pharmacotherapy. Prior use of psychotropic agents enhanced perceptions of their efficacy; prior illicit drug use did not influence their attitudes.

Family

Families must become involved in the entry phase during assessment, in the treatment phase, and in the discharge planning phase (James 1999). Some authors (Lewis et al. 1979) have described a higher prevalence of perinatal difficulties and bodily injuries, including head and facial physical trauma, in the early life of abused versus nonabused incarcerated youth. Therefore, systematic solicitation of early developmental history is an essential component of the assessment process. The family also has a major role in the psychological reconstitution of the youth, despite the fact that while in custody youths have limited interaction with their families. Parental reactions and emotional support can be powerful mediators of the child's symptoms.

Families can become active by monitoring symptoms and learning stress management techniques. Family intervention is also recommended because corroboration of symptoms is desirable. Family involvement also provides an opportunity for educating family members about psychotropic medications, the course of PTSD, and comorbid conditions. Once the youth is reunited with his or her family, a series of strategies that includes parental oversight and increasing youth accountability (James 1999) in collaboration with juvenile justice may be appropriate.

Violence in the home may precipitate traumatic responses among several family members. Clinicians may need to refer family members for additional individual treatment.

School, Detention Facilities, and Other Institutions

Youth can be approached at school or in detention facilities as described in the foregoing group treatment section. In addition, these sites provide the opportunity to educate school and probation staff about PTSD and relevant comorbid conditions and to develop collaborative strategies to assist youth in recovery. Triaging of school and institutional staff can also be done in these settings. Interventions may then be similarly provided on site.

Community System

Most youths return to their communities of origin and may remain in their communities while under delinquency court supervision. Efforts to provide community-based rehabilitation, including psychiatric rehabilitation, should be a multisystemic approach. These youth are involved with several systems including education, probation, mental health, and health, among others.

A forum for criminal justice and mental health experts was convened by the Substance Abuse and Mental Health Services Agency and the Department of Justice in 1999 to develop strategies to improve services to people with mental disorders who are in the justice system (U.S. Department of Justice 2000). Recommendations for juvenile justice and mental health included developing community programs, which included a research paradigm to evaluate effectiveness; developing statutes that compel youth and families to accept treatment when necessary; developing community programming that includes alternative treatments responsive to youth and family needs; and providing services that are culturally competent given the racial/ethnic diversity of youth in the juvenile justice system. Recommendations for detention facilities included identifying youth with mental disorders early in order to initiate care early; developing a transition process for those youth as they enter the adult system; providing training on mental illness for all custodial staff in detention facilities; and instituting federal oversight of detention facilities to ensure that adequate treatment is provided. Recommendations for interagency collaboration included integrating state juvenile justice systems with state mental health agencies; establishing partnerships among all child service agencies including but not limited to juvenile justice, child welfare, mental health, education, and health; consolidating public funding streams of substance abuse treatment and mental health treatment; establishing a continuum of care for these youth; and developing community and appropriate diversion alternatives to incarceration for youth with mental disorders. The incorporation of the Multi-Systemic Therapy Model (Henggler and Borduin 1990), which includes an in-home service component, into community-based efforts has demonstrated great promise.

Special programming for females (Cauffman et al. 1998; U.S. Department of Justice 2000) in detention facilities, especially those with mental disorders, should also be developed. Detention facilities and relevant programming have traditionally been designed for male detainees.

Remedial education is a key to community reintegration. Symptoms of PTSD in children and youth are known to jeopardize academic progress (Giaconia 1995). The high rate of PTSD among the incarcerated population coupled with comorbid learning disabilities (Barnum et al. 1989) may have very dire implications for the education of youth in the juvenile justice system.

Although many youths in custody may be involved in gangs, providing assistance to them so that they may change their patterns of risk behavior is critical. This may be more so with those youths who are particularly interested in avoiding the socially toxic environments in which they were raised. The juvenile justice system should collaborate with formerly incarcerated youth who have adopted a prosocial trajectory and have successfully reintegrated themselves into their communities. These youth could be valuable role models to those who struggle to leave gangs.

A substantial number of youths in the juvenile justice system are parents of very young children. Family planning and parenting instruction would be indicated for purposes of primary prevention, thereby minimizing the adverse impact on their very young offspring. A recent report (Greenwood et al. 1998) indicated that early childhood intervention strategies, parent education, high school monetary graduation incentives, and community-based supervision will likely decrease future crime rates and be cost effective.

Incarceration of juveniles in adult facilities predisposes them to further risk for victimization and therefore should be minimized if not completely eliminated.

Special National Challenge

A broader social and community problem is the significant racial and ethnic disparity in the confinement of juvenile offenders, an issue that has been the subject of politically contentious debates for at least several years. Of the incarcerated subjects with PTSD in the four studies discussed previously, 81% were of African American and Hispanic backgrounds. The Juvenile Justice and Delinquency Prevention Act of 1974 was amended by Congress in 1992 to establish the "disproportionate confinement of minority youth requirement," which mandated states that receive funding from the U.S. Department of Justice to determine the existence and extent of this problem statewide and demonstrate efforts to reduce it where it exists. Noncompliance with this requirement, along with three other "core requirements," could jeopardize their funding.

In 1997, children from minority backgrounds accounted for nearly 33% of the juvenile population nationwide but accounted for approximately two-thirds of the detained and committed population in secure detention facilities (Snyder and Sickmund 1999). African-American youths, despite accounting for only 15% of the juvenile population ages 10–17, accounted for 26% of the juveniles arrested and 45% of delinquency cases involving detention. Nearly 33% of adjudicated cases involved African-American youths, but 40% of juveniles in secure residential placements were African-American.

The reauthorization of the Juvenile Justice Delinquency and Prevention Act has been stymied in Congress for the past 3 years. Failure to pass this act may undermine the efforts by states to address and resolve this pattern of confinement and the perpetuation of confinement of minority youth from impoverished backgrounds whose families have historically had limited access to community services, including mental health services.

Summary

Many youths in the juvenile justice system have been exposed to myriad traumatic events, either as victims or as witnesses, since early childhood. These events are often associated with functional impairment in more than one key domain for varying periods of time. In addition, many such youths have developed PTSD, among other mental disorders, because of this exposure, thereby jeopardizing their development.

These youths, especially those committed to secure detention facilities, require mental health evaluations that specifically address victimization beginning from birth. Mental health interventions must go beyond addressing externalizing behaviors for which a youth may have been detained and confined. Mood disorders and substance abuse problems should also be a focus of care. Family participation is essential for effective mental health interventions.

Service system changes and paradigms, which promote an integrated service delivery approach, are critical for comprehensive rehabilitation of these youth. Research in this arena remains in a nascent phase and warrants more focus in the areas of epidemiology, natural course of PTSD for different age groups, protective factors relevant to PTSD, community factors, comorbidity, and effective mental health interventions (including pharmacologic interventions and family-oriented interventions).

References

Ahmad A, Mohammed K: The socioemotional development of orphans in orphanages and traditional foster care in Iraqi Kurdistan. Child Abuse Negl 20:1161–1173, 1996

Allen JA, Rappoport JL, Swedo SE: Psychopharmacologic treatment of childhood anxiety disorders, in Child and Adolescent Psychiatric Clinics of North America: Anxiety Disorders. Edited by Leonard HL, Philadelphia, PA, WB Saunders, 1993, pp 795–818

American Academy of Child and Adolescent Psychiatry: Practice Parameters for the Assessment and Treatment of Children and Adolescents with posttraumatic stress disorder. J Am Acad Child Adolesc Psychiatry 37(suppl):4S–26S, 1998

American Psychiatric Association: Diagnostic and Statistical Manual of Mental Disorders, 3rd Edition Revised. Washington, DC, American Psychiatric Association, 1987

American Psychiatric Association: Diagnostic and Statistical Manual of Mental Disorders, 4th Edition. Washington, DC, American Psychiatric Association, 1994

Arroyo W, Eth S: Children traumatized by Central American warfare, in Post-Traumatic Stress Disorders in Children. Edited by Eth S, Pynoos R. Washington, DC, American Psychiatric Press, 1985, pp 103–120

Arroyo W, Eth S: Post-traumatic stress disorder and other stress reactions, in Minefields in Their Hearts: the Mental Health of Children in War and Communal Violence. Edited by Apfel RJ, Simon B. New Haven, CT, University Press, 1996, pp 53–75

Arseneault J, Tremblay RE, Boulerice B, et al: Minor physical anomalies and family adversity as risk factors for violent delinquency in adolescence. Am J Psychiatry 157:917–923, 2000

Atkins DL, Pumariega AJ, Rogers K, et al: Mental health and incarcerated youth, I: prevalence and nature of psychopathology. Journal of Child and Family Studies 8:193–204, 1999

Barnum R, Famularo R, Bunshaft D, et al: Clinical evaluation of juvenile delinquents: who gets court referred? Bull Am Acad Psychiatry Law 17:335–344, 1989

Berliner L: Intervention with children who experience trauma, in The Effects of Trauma and the Developmental Process. Edited by Cicchetti D, Toth S. New York, Wiley, 1997, pp 491–514

Biederman J: Clonazepam in the treatment of prepubertal children with panic-like symptoms. J Clin Psychiatry 48(supp):38–42, 1987

Brady K, Pearlstein T, Asnis GM, et al: Efficacy and safety of sertraline treatment of posttraumatic stress disorder: a randomized controlled trial. JAMA 12:1837–1844, 2000

Brandenburg NA, Friedman RM, Silver SE: The epidemiology of childhood psychiatric disorders: prevalence findings from recent studies. J Am Acad Child Adolesc Psychiatry 29:76–83, 1990

Breslau N, Davis GC, Adreski P, et al: Traumatic events and posttraumatic stress disorder in an urban population of young adults. Arch Gen Psychiatry 48:216–222, 1991

Breton JJ, Valla JP, Lambert J: Industrial disaster and mental health of children and their parents. J Am Acad Child Adolesc Psychiatry 32:438–445, 1993

Burton D, Foy D, Bwanausi C, et al: The relationship between traumatic exposure, family dysfunction, and posttraumatic stress symptoms in male juvenile offenders. J Trauma Stress 7:83–93, 1994

Butterfield F: Prisons replace hospitals for the nation's mentally ill. New York Times, 5 March 1998, A1

Cauffman E, Feldman SS, Waterman J, et al: Posttraumatic stress disorder among female juvenile offenders. J Am Acad Child Adolescent Psychiatry, 37:1209–16, 1998

Center for Mental Health Services: 1998 Inventory of Mental Health Services in Juvenile Justice Facilities, Halfway Houses, and Group Homes Survey. Rockville, MD, U.S. Department of Health and Human Services, 1998

Cocozza JJ, Ingalls RP: Characteristics of Children in Out of Home Care. Albany, NY, New York State Council on Children and Families, 1984

Cocozza JJ, Skowyra KR: Youth with mental disorders: issues and emerging responses. Juvenile Justice 8:3–13, 2000

Davidson J, Kudler H, Smith R, et al: Treatment of post-traumatic stress disorder with amitryptaline and placebo. Arch Gen Psychiatry 47:259–266, 1990

Davidson JRT, Hughes D, Blazer DG, et al: Post traumatic stress disorder in the community: an epidemiological study. Psychol Med 21:713–721, 1991

Deblinger E, Heflin AH: Cognitive Behavioral Interventions for Treating Sexually Abused Children. Thousand Oaks, CA, Sage Publications, 1996

Dembo R, Williams L, Schmeidler J: Gender differences in mental health service needs. J Prison Jail Health 12:73–101, 1993

DiNicola VF: Ethnocentric aspects of posttraumatic stress disorder and related disorders among children and adolescents, in Ethnocultural Aspects of Posttraumatic Stress Disorders: Issues, Research, and Clinical Applications. Edited by Marsella J, Friedman MH, Gerrity ET, et al. Washington, DC, American Psychological Press, 1996, pp 389–414

Ditton PM: Mental health and treatment of inmates and probationers: special report. Washington, DC, U.S. Department of Justice, 1999

Dyregrov A, Gupta L, Gjestad R, et al: Trauma exposure and psychological reactions to genocide among Rwandan children. J Trauma Stress 13:3–21, 2000

Eth S, Pynoos R: Developmental perspective on psychic trauma in childhood, in Trauma and Its Wake. Edited by Figley CR. New York, NY, Brunner/Mazel, 1985, pp 36–52

Eth S, Arroyo W, Silverstein S: School consultation following the Los Angeles riots. Paper presented at the annual meeting of the American Psychiatric Association, San Francisco, CA, May 1993

Finkelhor D, Dziuba-Leatherman J: Victimization of children. Am Psychol 49:173–183, 1994

Fitzpatrick KM, Boldizar JP: The prevalence and consequences of exposure to violence among African-American youth. J Am Acad Child Adolescent Psychiatry 32:424–430, 1993

Foy DW, Madvig BT, Pynoos RS, et al: Etiologic factors in the development of posttraumatic stress disorder in children and adolescents. J School Psychol 34:133–145, 1996

Foy D, Wood JL, King DW, et al: Los Angeles Symptom Checklist: psychometric evidence with an adolescent sample. Assessment 4:377–383, 1997

Frank JB, Giller EL, Kosten TR, et al: A randomized clinical trial of phenelzine and imipramine for post-traumatic stress disorder. Am J Psychiatry 145:1289–1291, 1988

Friedman RM, Katz-Leavy JW, Manderscheid RW, et al: Prevalence of serious emotional disturbances in children and adolescents, in Mental Health, United States. Edited by Mandrscheid RW, Sonnerschein MA. Washington, DC, U.S. Department of Health and Human Services, 1996, pp 71–89

Galante R, Foa D: An epidemiological study of psychic trauma and treatment effectiveness for children after a natural disaster. J Am Acad Child Psychiatry 25:357–363, 1986

Garbarino J, Kostelny K: The effects of political violence on Palestinian children's behavior problems: a risk accumulation model. Child Development 67:33–45, 1996

Garrison CZ, Weinrich MW, Hardin SB, et al: Post-traumatic stress disorder in adolescents after a hurricane. Am J Epidemiol 138:522–530, 1993

Giaconia RM, Reinherz HZ, Silverman AB, et al: Traumas and posttraumatic stress disorder in a community population of older adolescents. J Am Acad Child Adolesc Psychiatry, 34:1369–1380, 1995

Goenjian AK, Pynoos RS, Steinberg AM, et al: Psychiatric co-morbidity in children after the 1988 earthquake in Armenia. J Am Acad Child Adolesc Psychiatry 34:1174–1184, 1995

Greenwood PW, Model KE, Rydell CP, et al: Diverting Children from a Life of Crime: Measuring the Costs and Benefits. Santa Monica, CA, Rand Publications, 1998

Grisso T, Barnum R: Massachusetts Youth Screening Instrument-2: User's Manual and Technical Report. Worcester, MA, University of Massachusetts Medical School, 2000

Halikas JA, Meller J, Morse C, et al: Predicting substance abuse in juvenile offenders: attention deficit disorder vs. aggressivity. Child Psychiatry and Human Development 21:49–55, 1990

Helzer JE, Robins LN, McEvoy L: Post-traumatic stress disorder in the general population. N Engl J Med 317:1630–1634, 1987

Henggler SW, Borduin CM: Family Therapy and Beyond: A Multisystemic Approach to Treating the Behavior Problems of Children and Adolescents. Pacific Grove, CA, Brooks/Cole, 1990

Herman J: Trauma and Recovery. New York, Basic Books, 1992

Hollander HE, Turner FD: Characteristics of incarcerated delinquents: relationship between development disorders, environmental and family factors, and patterns of offense and recidivism. J Amer Acad Child Psychiatry 24:221–226, 1985

Horowitz K, Weine S, Jekel J: PTSD symptoms in urban adolescent girls: compounded community trauma. J Am Acad Child Adolesc Psychiatry 34:1353–1361, 1995

Institute of Medicine: Research on Children and Adolescents with Mental, Behavioral and Development Disorders: Mobilizing a National Initiative. Washington, DC, National Academy Press, 1989

James CB: The Incarcerated Youth Needs Assessment Survey. Los Angeles, CA, Charles Drew University, 1999

Kinzie JD, Leung P: Clonidine in Cambodian patients with post-traumatic stress disorder. J Nerv Ment Dis 177:546–550, 1989

Kiser LJ, Ackerman BJ, Brown E, et al: Post-traumatic stress disorder in young children: a reaction to perpetual sexual abuse. J Am Acad Child Adolesc Psychiatry 27:645–649, 1988

Knitzer J: Juvenile justice and mental health: the forgotten mandate, in Unclaimed Children: The Failure of Public Responsibility to Children and Adolescents in Need of Mental Health Services. Edited by Knitzer J. Washington, DC, Children's Defense Fund, 1982

Kolb LC, Burris BC, Griffiths S: Propranolol and clonidine in the treatment of post-traumatic stress disorders of war, in Post-Traumatic Stress Disorder: Psychological and Biological Sequelae. Washington, DC, American Psychiatric Press, 1984

Kutcher SP, Reiter S, Gardner DM, et al: The Pharmacotherapy of Anxiety Disorders in Children and Adolescents. Psychiatr Clin North Am 15:41–66, 1992

Lewis DO, Shanok SS, Balla DA: Perinatal difficulties, head and face trauma, and child abuse in the medical histories of seriously delinquent children. Am J Psychiatry 136:419–423, 1979

Lucas AR, Pasley FC: Psychoactive drugs in the treatment of emotionally disturbed children: haloperidol and diazepam. Comprehensive Psychiatry 110:376–386, 1969

Myers WC, Scott K, Burgess AW, et al: Psychopathology, biopsychosocial factors, crime characteristics, and classification of 25 homicidal youths. J Am Acad Child Adolesc Psychiatry 34:1483–1489, 1995

Nader K, Pynoos R, Fairbanks L, et al: Children's PTSD reactions one year after a sniper attack at their school. Am J Psychiatry 147:1526–1530, 1990

Otto RK, Greenstein JJ, Johnson MK, et al: Prevalence of mental disorders among youth in the juvenile justice system, in Responding to the Mental Health Needs of Youth in the Juvenile Justice System. Edited by Cocozza JJ, Seattle, WA, National Coalition for the Mentally Ill in the Criminal Justice System, 1992, pp 7–48

Perry BD: Neurobiological sequelae of childhood trauma: PTSD in children, in Catecholamine Function in Posttraumatic Stress Disorder: Emerging Concepts. Edited by Murburg MM. Washington, DC, American Psychiatric Press, 1994, pp 233–255

Pfefferbaum B: Posttraumatic stress disorder in children: a review of the past ten years. J Am Acad Child Adolesc Psychiatry 36:1503–1511, 1997

Putnam FW: Dissociation in Children and Adolescents: A Developmental Perspective. New York, Guilford, 1997

Pynoos R, Eth S: Witness to violence: the child interview. J Am Acad Child Psychiatry 25:306–319, 1986

Pynoos RS, Nader K: Prevention of psychiatric morbidity in children after disaster, in OSAP Prevention Monograph-2 Prevention of Mental Disorders, Alcohol and Other Drug Use in Children and Adolescents (DHHS Publication ADM 899–1646). Edited by Shaffer D, Philips I, Enzer NB. Washington DC, U.S. Government Printing Office, 1989, pp 225–271

Pynoos RS, Nader K: Issues in the treatment of posttraumatic stress in children and adolescents, in International Handbook of Traumatic Stress Syndromes. Edited by Wilson JP, Raphael B. New York, Plenum, 1993, pp 535–549

Pynoos RS, Frederick C, Nader K, et al: Life threat and post-traumatic stress in school-age children. Arch Gen Psychiatry 44:1057–1063, 1987

Resnick HS, Kilpatrick DG, Dansky BS, et al: Prevalence of civilian trauma and post traumatic stress disorder in a representative national sample of women. J Consult Clin Psychol 61:984–991, 1993

Richters JE, Martinez P: The NIMH community violence project, I: children as victims and witnesses to violence. Psychiatry 56:7–21, 1993

Riddle MA, Bernstein GA, Cook EH, et al: Anxiolytics, adrenergic agents and naltrexone. J Am Acad Child Adolesc Psychiatry 38:546–556, 1999

Robbins DM, Beck JC, Pries R, et al: Learning disability and neuropsychological impairment in adjudicated, unincarcerated male delinquents. J Am Acad Child Adolescent Psychiatry 22:40–46, 1983

Romo C: Special report: short-changed, juvenile halls provide limited services because of inadequate resources. Los Angeles Daily Journal, 6 April 2000

Rosenbaum SH: Remarks by Chief, Special Litigation Section, Civil Rights Division, U.S. Department of Justice. 14th Annual National Juvenile Corrections and Detention Forum, Long Beach, CA, 1999

Schwab-Stone ME, Ayers TS, Wesley K, et al: No safe haven: a study of violence exposure in an urban community. J Am Acad Child Adolescent Psychiatry 34:1343–1352, 1995

Schwarz ED, Kowalski JM: Malignant memories: PTSD in children and adults after a school shooting. J Am Acad Child Adolesc Psychiatry 30:936–944, 1991

Smykla JO, Willis TW: The incidence of learning disabilities and mental retardation in youth under the jurisdiction of the juvenile court. Journal of Criminal Justice 9:219–225, 1981

Snyder HN, Sickmund M: Juvenile Offenders and Victims: 1999 National Report. Washington, DC, U.S. Department of Justice, 1999

Society for Adolescent Medicine: Health care for incarcerated youth: position paper of the Society for Adolescent Medicine. Journal of Adolescent Health 27:73–75, 2000

Stein A, Lewis DO: Discovering physical abuse: insights from a follow-up study of delinquents. Child Abuse Negl 16:523–531, 1992

Steiner H, Garcia I, Matthews Z: Posttraumatic stress disorder in incarcerated juvenile delinquents. J Am Acad Child Adolescent Psychiatry 36:357–365, 1997

Teplin LA: The prevalence of severe mental disorder among male urban jail detainees: comparison with the epidemiological catchment area program. Am J Public Health 80:663–669, 1990

Terr L: Treating psychic trauma in children: a preliminary discussion. J Trauma Stress 2:3–20, 1989

Terr L: Childhood traumas: an outline and overview. Am J Psychiatry 148:10–20, 1991

Thomas C, Holzer CE, Wall J: The Island Youth Programs: community interventions for reducing youth violence and delinquency. Adolescent Psychiatry, in press

Timmons-Mitchell J, Brown C, Schulz SC, et al: Comparing the mental health needs of female and male incarcerated juvenile delinquents. Behavior Sciences and the Law 15:195–202, 1997

U.S. Department of Justice: Executive summary of conference proceedings, in People with Mental Disorders in the Justice System: Strategies for Building on What We Know (July 22–23, 1999). Washington, DC, U.S. Department of Justice, 2000, pp 46–50

Widom CS, Ames MA: Criminal consequences of childhood sexual victimization. Child Abuse Negl 18:303–318, 1994

Williams RA, Hollis HM, Benoit K: Attitudes toward psychiatric medications among incarcerated female adolescents. J Am Acad Child Adolesc Psychiatry 37:1301–1307, 1998

Yehuda R, McFarlane AC: Conflict between current knowledge about posttraumatic stress disorder and its original conceptual basis. Am J Psychiatry 152:1705–1713, 1995

Chapter 4

Biological Treatment of PTSD in Children and Adolescents

Soraya Seedat, M.B.
Dan J. Stein, M.B.

Children and adolescents may develop posttraumatic stress disorder (PTSD) in the immediate or delayed aftermath of a traumatic event. Community studies in adolescents and young adults have reported trauma exposure rates (DSM-III-R; American Psychiatric Association 1987) ranging from 39% to 84% (Breslau et al. 1991; Vrana and Lauterbach 1994), whereas studies of at-risk children have yielded PTSD prevalence rates of between 3% and 100% (Garrison et al. 1995; Frederick 1985; Perkonigg et al. 2000). In a community sample of adolescents, 43% had experienced at least one DSM-III-R trauma by 18 years of age, and PTSD was evident in 14.5% of those exposed (Giaconia et al. 1995).

Although PTSD occurs in the context of exposure to an external high-magnitude stressor, these data demonstrate that not all children exposed to trauma develop PTSD; rather, it remains a complex disorder that is mediated by a range of biologic and psychologic factors. Biologic dysregulation of noradrenergic, serotonergic, glutamergic, and neuroendocrine pathways, among others, may play a role. The severity and duration of trauma exposure, physical and emotional proximity, individual patient characteristics, and parental factors may influence the develop-

The authors are supported by the Medical Research Council of South Africa.

ment of PTSD in children (Foy et al. 1996; Pfefferbaum 1997; Silva et al. 2000). Also, events that children report as particularly upsetting are not always the most likely to lead to PTSD. As is common with other psychiatric disorders, gender effects are evident in exposure to trauma and PTSD: girls have higher rates of trauma exposure and PTSD (Breslau et al. 1997; Cuffe et al. 1998; Giaconia et al. 1995) and different vulnerabilities to specific traumas (e.g., assaultive violence) compared with boys (Breslau et al. 1997, 1998; Kessler et al. 1995).

The presence of psychobiologic dysfunction in PTSD provides the clinician with a target for pharmacotherapeutic intervention (Friedman and Southwick 1995). However, the decision to begin a medication and the assessment of its efficacy require attention to the context within which the trauma has taken place and to the overall response of the child. In this chapter we review current knowledge of biologic treatments for child and adolescent PTSD, briefly addressing topics that are also relevant to pharmacotherapy, such as biologic dysregulation, symptom assessment, and the need for an integrative biopsychosocial approach to treatment.

Diagnosis and Phenomenology

The hallmark features of PTSD include a history of exposure to an index event that threatens the life or physical integrity of the person or others and the temporal development of symptoms from each of three symptom categories: reexperiencing of the trauma, avoidance and numbing, and hyperarousal (American Psychiatric Association 1994). This exposure induces a response in the child of intense fear, helplessness, or horror. For a diagnosis of PTSD, symptoms must cause significant distress and/or functional impairment and persist for longer than 1 month. The disorder runs a longitudinal course, with progressive modification of symptoms occurring over time (Blank 1993; McFarlane 2000).

Although the applicability of DSM-IV (American Psychiatric Association 1994) nosologic criteria to very young children is controversial, particularly as symptoms are often heterogenous and developmentally determined (Nader et al. 1990; Perry 1994; Weisenberg et al. 1993), these criteria provide a useful framework for guiding the assessment and treatment of PTSD in older children and adolescents (American Academy of Child and Adolescent Psychiatry 1998; Perrin et al. 2000). Certainly, the frequency and severity of symptoms in the three symptom clusters constitute a primary target for pharmacotherapy, and these symptoms should be carefully monitored during treatment.

Important differences in clinical presentation may exist between acute (duration of symptoms less than 3 months) and chronic (duration of symptoms 3 months or more) subtypes in children. Famularo et al. (1996), for example, described prominent reexperiencing, hyperarousal, and sleep difficulties in the acute subtype and detachment, restricted affect, dissociation, and depressed mood in the chronic subtype. A two-tiered classification of childhood traumas has been proposed by Terr (1991): Type I (single-incident, sudden, characterized by detailed memories and misperceptions) and Type II (chronic, recurrent, usually childhood physical and/or sexual abuse, characterized by denial, numbing, dissociation, and/or rage). These subtypes may be mediated by different psychobiologic factors and may require different treatment approaches (Donnelly et al. 1999). For example, symptom targets in patients with more chronic PTSD may, in addition to the core symptom clusters, need to include symptoms such as guilt and shame. Also, medications that theoretically decrease the ability of patients to respond to the psychotherapeutic interventions aimed at resolving these issues (Gelpin et al. 1996; Risse et al. 1990) may be relatively contraindicated.

Childhood PTSD also precedes, predisposes the patient to, and co-occurs with other psychiatric disorders. Although studies investigating the time sequencing of PTSD and comorbid conditions have yielded conflicting results, the high rates of comorbidity with mood, anxiety, and substance use disorders are comparable with those for adults and may have a significant impact on prevention and treatment (Brady 1997; Famularo et al. 1992; Deykin and Buka 1997; Giaconia et al. 1995; Goenjian et al. 1995; Green 1985; Hubbard et al. 1995; Kessler et al. 1995; McCloskey and Walker 2000; Yehuda and McFarlane 1995). Children with comorbid disorders, such as depressive and anxiety disorders, require interventions with broad-spectrum effects. In addition, certain medications (e.g., benzodiazepines) may be relatively contraindicated for patients with comorbid substance use disorders.

Furthermore, children with PTSD have been shown to have more behavioral, emotional, and interpersonal problems; academic failures; suicidal behaviors; and health problems than those without PTSD (Giaconia et al. 1995; Mazza 2000; Schwab-Stone et al. 1999). Although clinical trials in the past have focused on issues of efficacy and tolerability, there is increasing recognition of the need to focus on the effectiveness of pharmacotherapy in day-to-day practice. Patients who are eligible for entry into clinical trials may represent a particular subgroup of patients; those with milder and more severe PTSD (e.g., with suicidal ideation or substantial comorbidity) may be excluded from trials, thus limiting the generalizability of findings. Moreover, the focus in clinical trials to date has been on core PTSD symptoms rather than on determining whether pharmacotherapy is useful in addressing broader quality-of-life issues.

Neurobiologic Systems in PTSD

Accumulated evidence indicates that severe psychologic trauma may effect chronic alterations in the neurobiology of the stress response (Bremner et al. 1993; Charney et al. 1993; De Bellis et al. 1994; Heim et al. 2000). Models of "fear-conditioning" (Le Doux 1996) have been particularly useful in exploring the psychobiology of PTSD. These models implicate the amygdala and other regions of the limbic system and also suggest that several neurochemical systems are likely to be relevant, including the noradrenergic, serotonergic, glutamergic, GABAergic, dopaminergic, opioid, hypothalamic-pituitary-adrenal, hypothalamic-pituitary-thyroid, hypothalamic-pituitary-growth hormone, and hypothalamic-pituitary-gonadal systems. We review some of the relevant findings in the sections below.

Advances in structural and functional imaging in PTSD patients have provided further information about the neuroanatomy of PTSD. A network of brain regions, comprising the amygdala, hippocampus, anterior cingulate, Broca's area, and visual cortex, has been implicated (De Bellis et al. 2000; Hamner et al. 1999). Although much of the original work was done in adults, there is a growing body of literature concerning children and adolescents. In a recently published magnetic resonance imaging study (De Bellis et al. 1999a, 1999b), maltreated children and adolescents with PTSD demonstrated smaller intracranial and cerebral volumes than matched controls but not the predicted decrease in hippocampal volume seen in adult PTSD (Stein et al. 1997). Also, brain volume correlated robustly and positively with the age of onset of PTSD but correlated negatively with the duration of abuse.

Neuroendocrine Alterations

Converging evidence supports the hypothesis that alterations of the hypothalamic-pituitary-adrenal axis in PTSD are different from those in acute and chronic stress and major depression. These are conditions associated with both increased corticotropin releasing factor (CRF) and cortisol levels. Although CRF levels are increased in PTSD, findings include 1) paradoxically low ambient cortisol levels (Holsboer et al. 1984; Yehuda 1998); 2) an increased sensitivity of the hypothalamic-pituitary-adrenal axis to negative feedback inhibition (Yehuda et al. 1993, 1995); 3) increased concentration and sensitivity of lymphocyte glucocorticoid receptors (Yehuda et al. 1993); and 4) an augmented adrenocorticotropin response to metyrapone administration (Yehuda et al. 1996). Findings of low urinary cortisol levels have been supported by plasma and salivary cortisol levels. In a study examining adult urinary cortisol levels in children of Holocaust survivors, low cortisol levels were present in those who had PTSD as well as those who had not been exposed to traumatic events and had no PTSD but whose parents had PTSD. Thus, low cortisol levels characterized children with the specific risk factor of parental PTSD (Yehuda et al. 2000).

Goenjian et al. (1996) demonstrated that basal salivary cortisol levels were lower in adolescents who had been closer to the epicenter of the Armenian earthquake 5 years earlier and who still had substantial PTSD symptoms compared with children who had been farther away from the epicenter and who, as a group, had fewer symptoms. De Bellis et al. (1999a, 1999b) reported that maltreated prepubertal children with PTSD excreted higher concentrations of 24-hour urinary free cortisol and had significantly higher concentrations of urinary dopamine and norepinephrine than did those with overanxious disorder and control subjects. Urinary free cortisol and urinary catecholamine concentrations also showed a positive correlation with duration of trauma and severity of PTSD symptoms, suggesting that maltreatment experiences are associated with alterations of biologic stress systems in these patients.

CRF antagonists are being investigated as a treatment for depression and possibly PTSD. Presumably, a reduction in CRF activity in patients would cause cortisol levels to fall, thus reducing the increased sensitivity of the hypothalamic-pituitary-adrenal axis to negative feedback.

Neurotransmitter Systems

Norepinephrine

The finding that stress produces marked increases in brain noradrenergic function and that fear conditioning is mediated by alterations in noradrenergic activity may be important in understanding the pathophysiology of PTSD (Charney et al. 1993). Many of the symptoms experienced in PTSD, such as panic attacks, insomnia, exaggerated startle, and autonomic hyperarousal, are characteristic of increased noradrenergic function. Drugs like opiates and benzodiazepines either attenuate or decrease the stress-induced increases in norepinephrine release (Charney et al. 1993). Yohimbine has been used as a noradrenergic probe in combat veterans with PTSD to activate noradrenergic neurons (by blocking the presynaptic α_2-adrenergic autoreceptor) (Southwick et al. 1997). More than 40% of these patients had yohimbine-induced panic attacks and had significantly greater increases in anxiety and PTSD symptoms compared with control subjects. Yohimbine's propensity to elicit flashbacks and traumatic memory in PTSD patients may relate to stimulation of β-adrenergic receptors in the amygdala and cortical structures (Cahil et al. 1994). It can be speculated that attenuation of noradrenergic activity with drugs, such as clonidine, that act presynaptically to decrease norepinephrine release may have clinical application in patients with PTSD (Nutt 2000).

Serotonin

Conditioned fear stimuli activate serotonergic neurons in the dorsal raphe nucleus, projecting to the amygdala and forebrain. Animal models of PTSD suggest that serotonergic pathways mediate certain avoidance behaviors, whereas clinical studies of paroxetine platelet binding and m-CPP challenge tests further suggest a role for serotonin in PTSD (Arora et al. 1993; Southwick et al. 1997). For example, m-CPP (M-chlorophenylpiperazine, a serotonin agonist) has been shown to induce panic attacks, flashbacks, and dissociative episodes in a significant number of combat veterans with PTSD compared with a control group (Southwick et al. 1997). In addition, patients who had panic attacks induced by m-CPP were not the same as those who had panic attacks induced by yohimbine, perhaps suggesting two distinct subgroups of PTSD patients, one with a sensitized serotonergic system and the other with a sensitized noradrenergic system. This finding, although not empirically tested in adults or children, suggests that it may ultimately be possible to use biologic markers to help choose pharmacologic interventions.

Dopamine

Acute stress increases dopamine release in the prefrontal cortex and may, in turn, be linked to specific PTSD symptoms, including panic attacks, hypervigilance, exaggerated startle, and generalized anxiety (Antelman 1988). A role for the dopaminergic system in PTSD is supported by observations that cocaine and amphetamines (which increase dopamine turnover) can produce hypervigilance and paranoia, and drugs that reduce dopaminergic function (such as dopamine blocking agents) may alleviate these effects.

Glutamate and GABA

There is a growing body of evidence supporting the role of glutamergic and GABA pathways in PTSD; these pathways are involved in the normal encoding of memory. Benzodiazepines and alcohol are known to potentiate the effects of GABA, and patients with PTSD frequently use these drugs to suppress or prevent the reemergence of previous memories (Nutt 2000).

Summary

Much remains unknown about the psychobiology of PTSD in children and adolescents. The plasticity of the brain in children may, on the one hand, be used to argue for a more conservative approach with regard to medication. On the other hand, the negative impact of PTSD symptoms on developmental maturation may be used to argue for early and rigorous pharmacologic interventions. Detailed study of the psychobiology of PTSD over time, and of the effects of pharmacotherapy on this psychobiology, is needed.

Biologic Treatments in Children and Adolescents

There is currently relatively little empirical research on the use of medications to treat children with PTSD (Donnelly et al. 1999; March et al. 1996). The literature that does exist is characterized primarily by anecdotal case reports and open trials of various pharmacologic agents. Pharmacologic agents that have been suggested and tried in children and adolescents with PTSD include propranolol (Famularo et al. 1988), clonidine (Harmon and Riggs 1996), guanfacine (Horrigan and Barnhill 1996), carbamazepine (Looff et al. 1995), tricyclic antidepressants (TCAs), and serotonergic agents (Pfefferbaum 1997). Most clinicians tend to rely heavily on clinical experience and extrapolation of data from adult populations to inform their choice of medications in this population.

Although a variety of psychosocial treatments have been employed, cognitive-behavioral treatment (CBT) approaches have the strongest empirical evidence for efficacy in both children and adults with PTSD and should arguably be considered as a first-line approach, either alone or in combination with other forms of treatment (American Academy of Child and Adolescent Psychiatry 1998). Although most forms of CBT incorporate exposure techniques, it has not yet been established how intense or how explicit exposure needs to be to effect a therapeutic response (March et al. 2000).

Furthermore, the exact value of medication strategies alone and in combination with psychosocial interventions is unclear (Allen et al. 1995; American Academy of Child and Adolescent Psychiatry 1998; Pfefferbaum 1997). In a retrospective case analysis of 76 patients presenting with PTSD to a child and adolescent unit, most patients were treated with both psychotherapy and medication (imipramine and fluoxetine were the medications most frequently prescribed). At discharge from hospital, 42.1% were rated as much improved or very much improved on the Clinical Global Impression (CGI) Scale (Guy 1976; Traut A, Kaminer D, Boshoff D, et al: "PTSD in an Inpatient Child and Adolescent Psychiatric Unit," unpublished data, 2000). Although medications can be argued to facilitate psychotherapy, there is the theoretical concern that some agents might not be effective in doing so. This is clearly an area in which further research is required.

Selective Serotonin Reuptake Inhibitors

Several large open and controlled studies of the selective serotonin reuptake inhibitors (SSRIs) in adult PTSD have demonstrated these compounds to be effective in this disorder. Studies in which these agents have proven more effective than placebo have focused on patients with noncombat PTSD and chronic PTSD (i.e., duration longer than 3 months). Sertraline was recently approved as the first drug treatment for adult PTSD. To date, however, there are no published controlled studies of SSRI use in children or adolescents with PTSD.

Two recent placebo-controlled studies of sertraline in adults with DSM-III-R chronic PTSD (duration at least 6 months) yielded significant efficacy for sertraline over placebo on all PTSD symptom clusters, with sertraline being well tolerated (Brady et al. 2000); 53% of patients were much improved or very much improved at treatment endpoint ($P=0.008$ versus placebo), with 70% of the reduction in PTSD symptom severity achieved within the first 4 weeks of treatment. The efficacy of sertraline was significant compared with that of placebo in reducing symptom severity for symptom clusters of arousal and avoidance/numbing but not for the reexperiencing symptoms.

In a 5-week study of fluoxetine in male and female veteran and civilian subjects ($n=64$), PTSD symptoms were significantly reduced from baseline in fluoxetine-treated patients relative to placebo (van der Kolk et al. 1994). In a 12-week double-blind study comparing fluoxetine (up to 60 mg/day) with placebo in civilians ($n=53$), 85% of patients receiving fluoxetine and 62% receiving placebo had a Duke Global Rating for PTSD (Davidson et al. 1998) improvement score of 1 or 2 (very much or much improved). In addition, a stricter definition of "good outcome" (based on interview, self-rating scales, and disability rating scales) was associated with a response rate of 41% for fluoxetine and 4% for placebo (Connor et al. 1999).

In the largest open trial of an SSRI in a noncombat population, paroxetine was effective for chronic DSM-III-R PTSD. Of note was that much of the improvement in hyperarousal and avoidance symptoms occurred in the first 8 weeks of treatment, with reexperiencing symptoms improving more gradually by week 12 (Marshall et al. 1998).

Open trials of fluvoxamine in combat veterans (Marmar et al. 1996) and civilians (Davidson et al. 1998) have also shown efficacy in treating PTSD symptoms. In a recently published study that assessed the effect of fluvoxamine in 16 adults with PTSD and 16 healthy matched control subjects exposed to trauma scripts, 10 weeks of fluvoxamine treatment (100–300 mg/day) significantly improved patients' PTSD, depression, and autonomic reactivity (heart rate and blood pressure) (Tucker et al. 2000).

To our knowledge, only one open trial of an SSRI in adolescents with PTSD has been published. In a small trial ($n=8$) of 12 weeks of citalopram treatment in adolescents with moderate to severe PTSD, all seven completers were rated as much improved or very much improved on the CGI Scale (Seedat et al., in press). Core PTSD symptoms (reexperiencing, avoidance, hyperarousal) showed statistically significant improvement at week 12 on the Clinician-Administered PTSD Scale Child and Adolescent Version (CAPS-CA; Nader et al. 1994). Citalopram was well tolerated, with reported adverse experiences being mild.

Given the lack of controlled trials of SSRIs (placebo controlled or using active comparators) and other medications in childhood PTSD, any recommendation can only be tentative. Nevertheless, there are several reasons for suggesting that SSRIs are a first-line agent of choice in this population. First, although extrapolation from adult data can be problematic, there is good evidence of the efficacy and tolerability of this class in older PTSD patients. Certainly, current consensus guidelines emphasize the role of the SSRIs in adult PTSD, a finding supported by a meta-analysis of six controlled studies of PTSD in adults that reported a correlation between greater serotonergic activity and higher effect size (Penava et al. 1997).

Second, the SSRIs have been found to be safe and effective in a range of mood and anxiety disorders in children and adolescents, and such disorders are commonly comorbid with PTSD. The safety profiles of the SSRIs are superior to those of the TCAs, and the SSRIs do not require the therapeutic drug monitoring required for TCAs (Preskorn et al. 1994). Moreover, SSRIs are relatively safe in overdose. This difference is particularly important in children, who are more susceptible to the toxic effects of TCAs than are adults because of the increased production of cardiotoxic metabolites of these drugs in this population (Leonard et al. 1997).

Tricyclic Antidepressants and Monoamine Oxidase Inhibitors

There are no randomized clinical trials of either the TCAs or monoamine oxidase inhibitors (MAOIs) in children with PTSD. In adults, double-blind data support the efficacy of the TCAs imipramine and amitriptyline (Davidson et al. 1990; Kosten et al. 1991). Desipramine, a more noradrenergic agent, was not effective, although this was only a 4-week study. This result supports findings that noradrenergic-specific agents are less effective than serotonergic-specific agents in adults with PTSD (Dow and Kline 1997; Penava et al. 1997). The noradrenergic agents might be particularly useful for targeting reexperiencing symptoms (e.g., intrusive memories, flashbacks).

TCAs have been shown in open-label trials and case reports to be effective in children and adolescents with panic disorder (Black and Robbins 1990; Garland and Smith 1990) and have also been shown to be effective in placebo-controlled trials of separation anxiety disorder and school refusal (Gittelman-Klein and Klein 1971). Furthermore, in the first prospective double-blind pilot study of imipramine and chloral hydrate treatment in acute stress disorder in 25 children (aged 2–19 years) who had sustained serious burns, imipramine was significantly more effective than chloral hydrate in treating acute stress disorder symptoms (Robert et al. 1999).

In view of safety concerns and a less favorable side effect profile, TCAs would be a second-line treatment, after the SSRIs, in child and adolescent PTSD. After all, side effects may not necessarily affect compliance. A recent 8-week double-blind study compared the side effects and medication compliance of imipramine with those of placebo, each in combination with CBT, in 63 anxious depressed adolescents with school refusal. Mean side effects were significantly higher for the imipramine group, but these were not associated with noncompliance (Bernstein et al. 2000).

Like the TCAs, the MAOIs (e.g., phenelzine and brofaromine) have also demonstrated efficacy in placebo-controlled trials in adults (Baker et al. 1995; Kosten et al. 1991). Because the irreversible MAOIs (e.g., phenelzine) necessitate dietary restrictions, and because of the risk of medical complications (e.g., hypertensive crises), the MAOIs are not regularly prescribed in children and adolescents. Moclobemide, the only available reversible inhibitor of MAO-A, was shown to be effective in an open-label trial of adult patients who met DSM-III-R criteria for PTSD (Neal et al. 1997), but has not been studied in children and adolescents with PTSD and is not available in the United States.

β-*Blockers and* α$_2$-*Agonists*

In adults, open-label propranolol (a β-blocker) given to combat veterans with PTSD ($n=12$) in a dose of 120–160 mg/day resulted in improvement in explosiveness, nightmares, sleep, startle response, and hyperalertness (Kolb et al. 1984). Similarly, Famularo et al. (1988) reported that propranolol (dose, 2.5 mg/kg) had positive effects in 11 sexually abused children following a 5-week course of treatment, particularly on symptoms of hypervigilance and hyperarousal.

Clonidine, an α_2-agonist, was initially considered to be potentially useful for attention-deficit/hyperactivity disorder (ADHD) symptoms in sexually abused children. It was also effective in children with comorbid PTSD (De Bellis et al. 1994; Marmar et al. 1993). Clonidine patches (0.1–0.2 mg/day) were subsequently administered to preschool children with PTSD and to children whose PTSD symptoms of impulsivity, aggression, and hyperarousal had not remitted with other treatments (Harmon and Riggs 1996). The use of clonidine patches in this open trial was observed to be better tolerated than that of oral clonidine and caused less sedation. Clonidine was effective in reducing hyperarousal, aggression, and sleep disturbance in children with severe PTSD. However, the authors cautioned that parental compliance was important because precipitous discontinuation of clonidine could be dangerous. Also, clonidine should be given together with close medical monitoring and only to children free of cardiac or other major medical illness. Additional drawbacks are the risk of hypotension and tolerance to the therapeutic effects with long-term use. Another α_2-agonist, guanfacine, which has a longer half-life than clonidine, was reported in a single case to be beneficial in reducing nightmares in a 7-year-old child with PTSD (Horrigan and Barnhill 1996).

Anticonvulsants

Anticonvulsants have been suggested for the treatment of PTSD based on the hypothesis that repeated trauma exposure can eventually lead to sensitization of limbic circuits and a lowering of the firing threshold (neuronal kindling) (Post and Kopanda 1976). This model may arguably be applicable to chronic child abuse (physical and sexual) or to the reexperiencing phenomena that might occur from a single trauma (van der Kolk et al. 1989). In adults with PTSD, benefits have been reported predominantly in open-label trials with carbamazepine (Lipper et al. 1986), sodium valproate (Fesler 1991), lamotrigine (Hertzberg et al. 1999), and gabapentin (Brannon et al. 2000).

Looff et al. (1995) reported on the effective use of carbamazepine in 28 children with PTSD (dose, 300–1,200 mg/day; serum levels, 10.0–11.5 µg/mL). In this study, 22 children had complete remission of symptoms, and the remaining 6 children were significantly improved on all other PTSD symptoms except nightmares related to ongoing abuse. These findings were confounded by multiple comorbid diagnoses in the sample (depression, ADHD, polysubstance abuse, oppositional defiant disorder) and by the fact that many children were receiving concomitant medications (imipramine, fluoxetine, sertraline, clonidine, methylphenidate).

Other Agents

Serotonergic Agents

Other serotonergic agents such as buspirone (a 5-HT_{1A} [5-hydroxytryptamine-1A] partial agonist) may be effective in treating some symptoms of PTSD (insomnia, nightmares, flashbacks, anxiety, and depressed mood) when used as monotherapy (LaPorta and Ware 1992; Wells et al. 1991) or as antidepressant augmentation (Hamner et al. 1997). Cyproheptadine, an antihistaminic 5-HT antagonist, has also been reported to be useful in relieving nightmares (Gupta et al. 1998). It has been suggested that because of its sedative action, cyproheptadine might be useful for sleep onset problems and nightmares in children with PTSD (Donnelly et al. 1999).

Similarly, nefazodone (a 5-HT_2 antagonist) and trazodone (Davidson et al. 1998; Davis et al. 1998; Hertzberg et al. 1996) have also been shown in open-label trials to be useful for sleep problems, aggression, and nightmares and may provide similar benefits in childhood PTSD. Nefazodone was recently reported to be particularly useful in adolescents with PTSD in addressing symptoms of hyperarousal, including anger, aggression, restlessness, insomnia, and even impaired concentration (Domon and Andersen 2000). Adolescents often reported an improvement in both sleep duration and sleep quality. In the context of residential treatment, the authors observed an improvement in avoidance, anhedonia, and detachment.

To our knowledge, there have been no controlled studies of these agents in children.

Opioid Antagonists

Opioid antagonists have yielded mixed results in adults with PTSD, but there is no published literature on their use in children or adolescents with PTSD. Disturbed opioid function has been hypothesized in PTSD, with the observation that naloxone (an opioid antagonist) reversed stress-induced analgesia in combat veterans with PTSD who were reexposed to trauma-related scenes (van der Kolk et al. 1989). In an open-label trial of the opioid antagonist nalmefene, Glover (1993) reported that 8 of 18 veterans had reduction in numbing symptoms, but many experienced worsening of other PTSD symptoms.

Benzodiazepines

Despite the use of benzodiazepines in PTSD, few studies have been performed in adults and none in children and adolescents with PTSD. Alprazolam and clonazepam have been shown to reduce anxiety and insomnia but have not been shown to have significant effects on the core PTSD symptom clusters (Braun et al. 1990; Lowenstein et al. 1988). Controlled studies of benzodiazepines for other childhood anxiety disorders (e.g., panic disorder, school refusal) have shown them to be superior to placebo (Bernstein et al. 1990; Kutcher et al. 1992).

Although benzodiazepines may be a useful adjunct to antidepressant treatments, their potential for dependence and other adverse effects makes them a less-than-ideal choice in this population. Theoretically, they may have a negative impact on behavioral therapy.

Dopamine Blocking Agents

The use of dopamine blocking agents in PTSD is not well defined. The classical antipsychotics have usually been reserved for very severe and/or treatment-refractory cases. Dillard et al. (1993), for example, reported on a combat veteran with severe flashbacks who responded to treatment with thioridazine. With the advent of the atypical agents (i.e., olanzapine, risperidone, quetiapine) and their lower risk of extrapyramidal side effects, there is likely to be more widespread use in PTSD. Risperidone has been successfully used in adults with PTSD to treat nightmares, flashbacks, irritability, intrusive thoughts, and aggression (Krashin and Oates 1999; Leyba and Wampler 1998; Monnelly and Ciraulo 1999).

The first open trial of risperidone (average dose, 1.3 mg/day for 16 weeks) conducted in adolescent boys with severe PTSD ($n=18$) showed significant improvement in 50%, moderate improvement in 22%, and mild improvement in 11% on the CGI Scale. Notably, comorbidity in the sample was high, with 83% meeting criteria for ADHD, 56% for oppositional defiant disorder, 33% for bipolar disorder, 22% for conduct disorder, and 11% for major depression. Only 11% met criteria for psychosis (Horrigan 1998). Nevertheless, some caution is required; there are, for example, reports of the development of tardive dyskinesia in an adolescent treated concurrently with risperidone (0.5 mg/day), methylphenidate (30 mg/day), and fluoxetine (20 mg/day) (Feeney and Klykylo 1996).

Lithium Carbonate

Lithium carbonate has been useful for symptoms of irritability, anger, and insomnia in open trials of adults (Forster et al. 1995; Kitchner and Greenstein 1985). There are no published data on its use in child and adolescent PTSD.

Augmentation Strategies

Augmentation strategies in PTSD have been poorly studied. Case studies and open trials have reported on the benefits of augmenting antidepressant response with clonidine (Kinzie and Leung 1989), anticonvulsants (Fesler 1991), and buspirone (Hamner et al. 1997) in adult PTSD. Gillette and Tannery (1994) described two cases of 9-year-old children with PTSD. Propranolol was added to imipramine treatment for control of anger, aggression, and impulsivity. Both patients experienced apparent inhibition of imipramine metabolism and near-toxic levels while receiving these medications. Competitive inhibition of imipramine metabolism can occur with coadministration of propranolol, resulting in a decreased clearance and increased half-life for imipramine.

Appropriate Treatment

The level of care (outpatient/inpatient) and treatment modality (pharmacotherapy, individual therapy, family therapy) should be tailored according to the individual child and the stage, course, and severity of the disorder (American Academy of Child and Adolescent Psychiatry 1998). Certainly, it is important to bear in mind that a recommendation to use medication may be interpreted in a range of different ways by the patient and family and that this issue should be explored. However, as with adult PTSD, it seems reasonable to make such a recommendation when symptoms are more severe, when there are comorbid mood and anxiety disorders, or when there is substantial disruption of functioning (Ballenger et al. 2000). A low-dose SSRI should be used at first, with the dose gradually titrated upward to the same (or higher) dose used to treat depression. An appropriate trial of initial drug therapy is 3 months. Effective pharmacotherapy should be continued for 12 months or longer, depending on the severity and duration of symptoms and impairment.

Predictors of Response to Pharmacotherapy

In adults, there is an emerging body of literature on the predictors of response to pharmacotherapy in PTSD. In an earlier trial of amitriptyline that focused on predictors of response in combat veterans, Davidson et al. (1993) reported that prior degree of combat intensity, current levels of PTSD, levels of depression and anxiety, symptoms of guilt, some avoidance symptoms, and the personality trait of neuroticism all predicted poor response to amitriptyline. In a more recent naturalistic follow-up study of fluoxetine treatment in adults with PTSD (Davidson 2000), predictors of outcome at 15 months were investigated, including baseline symptoms, gender, types of trauma, number of traumas, and clinical response in the first 2 weeks. Only one variable—how well patients had done in the first 3 months—was significant as a positive predictor of long-term outcome. In another study of pooled data from six trials of nefazodone involving both civilians and combat veterans, predictors of response to nefazodone at treatment endpoint included age, gender, and trauma type (Hidalgo et al. 1999). To date, there are no such studies in children and adolescents. The adult literature has indicated that combat veterans may have a poorer response to medication than civilians; it may be hypothesized that children who live in environments characterized by ongoing threat and who have less social support will have a poorer response to pharmacotherapy.

Recent developments in molecular biology and pharmacogenetics, particularly the exploration of how genetic polymorphisms influence individual vulnerabilities to trauma and illness as well as response to medication, may ultimately contribute to a more accurate delineation of treatment response predictors in PTSD.

Assessing Outcome in Children and Adolescents

When assessing children and adolescents with PTSD, clinicians mostly rely on direct interviewing of the child and parents. However, several semistructured interviews and parent/child self-report measures of PTSD symptoms have been developed to aid assessment. The PTSD Reaction Index (self-report) (Pynoos et al. 1987), which has a composite score to indicate the severity of PTSD symptoms, has been the most widely used measure in epidemiologic studies (Bradburn 1991; Goenjian et al. 1995; Nader et al. 1993; Shaw et al. 1995). With the advent of the Clinician-Administered PTSD Scale Child and Adolescent Version (CAPS-CA) (Nader et al. 1994), modeled on the adult CAPS, a reliable and valid current and lifetime DSM-IV diagnosis of PTSD can be generated in individuals ages 8 years through to adolescence. The CAPS-CA assesses both frequency and severity of each symptom as well as overall severity of PTSD and is likely to follow the adult CAPS as a widely used instrument in clinical trials. The Child PTSD Symptom Scale (CPSS) (Foa EB, Johnson K, Feeny NC, et al: "The Child PTSD Symptom Scale (CPSS): Validation of a Measure for Children with PTSD," unpublished data, 2000) is a newer instrument that also measures the severity of PTSD symptoms in children exposed to trauma. The psychometric properties of the CPSS show high internal consistency and test–retest reliability.

Extensive reliability and validity data on these instruments have yet to be made available. There is currently no "gold standard" for assessing PTSD treatment outcome (to medications or psychotherapies) in clinical trials of children and adolescents. A more global and informative instrument needs to be developed for use in pediatric clinical trials that will measure not only all symptom dimensions but also the extent of disability and quality of life. In addition, clinicians need to be aware of important symptoms in PTSD that fall outside the diagnostic criteria; for example, when issues of guilt, shame, mistrust, and dysfunctional interpersonal relationships are found, these ought to be monitored during treatment. On the other hand, there is a need to develop a standardized instrument that is brief and easy enough to administer in primary care and other settings in which patients with the disorder may be seen.

Quality of Life

Significant physical and medical problems in childhood, adolescence, and adulthood appear to be related to childhood trauma. There is a growing body of literature highlighting the long-term effects of trauma exposure and PTSD on physical health and use of medical services. PTSD is associated with higher rates of cardiovascular, gastrointestinal, respiratory, and neurologic complaints and more frequent visits to primary care practitioners (Boscarino and Chang 1999; Kessler et al. 1995; Shalev et al. 1990). The relationship among exposure to trauma, poor health, and greater use of health services has been established in adults, and although a neglected area of study, likely holds true for children.

Conclusions

Pharmacologic studies of PTSD in children have thus far lacked rigor in experimental design and assessment of efficacy. Ideally, for a medication to be considered effective, it should decrease symptoms across all three symptom clusters (intrusion, avoidance, and increased arousal), improve other symptoms such as aggression and impulsivity, treat comorbid disorders, and facilitate adjunctive psychosocial interventions (such as CBT).

Double-blind, randomized, placebo-controlled trials are needed to confirm observations of efficacy as are comparative studies of the efficacy of drug therapy, CBT, and a combination of the two approaches. More data are needed on the predictors of response to pharmacotherapy, optimum length of treatment, and rate of relapse on discontinuation as well as studies of children and adolescents with PTSD that is refractory to standard treatment.

It is important to provide more evidence-based criteria for initiating pharmacotherapy in children and to determine whether early intervention (e.g., during acute stress disorder) with medication has a beneficial effect on long-term outcome. Little is known about the impact of early intervention because most controlled trials have included patients who have chronic PTSD. Another area to explore is whether biologic markers such as cortisol, catecholamine, and heart rate predict illness development and/or response to treatment.

Ultimately, the duration of any treatment intervention must be determined in the clinical context of dose and time response. Additionally, the issue of differential drug effect on different PTSD subtypes needs to be addressed. Distinguishing between acute and chronic PTSD, for example, may potentially affect both the selection and duration of drug treatment.

Treatment of PTSD in children and adolescents, as with adults, should arguably be multimodal, but this recommendation too requires additional research. Because parental reactions can theoretically aid or hinder recovery, treatment plans should incorporate a family perspective.

Despite the many questions that remain for further study, there is a growing database on children and adolescents that suggests that medications should not be ignored. Medications may be useful not only in reducing core PTSD symptoms but also in addressing secondary and comorbid symptoms, in improving quality of life, and in supporting a healthy developmental course. In particular, the SSRIs may be a particularly useful intervention in childhood PTSD. This preliminary work deserves the attention of both clinicians and researchers.

References

Allen AJ, Leonard H, Swedo S: Current knowledge of medications for the treatment of childhood anxiety disorders. J Am Acad Child Adolesc Psychiatry 38:976–986, 1995

American Academy of Child and Adolescent Psychiatry: Practice parameters for the assessment and treatment of children and adolescents with posttraumatic stress disorder. J Am Acad Child Adolesc Psychiatry 37(suppl 10):4S–26S, 1998

American Psychiatric Association: Diagnostic and Statistical Manual of Mental Disorders, 3rd Edition Revised. Washington, DC, American Psychiatric Association, 1987

American Psychiatric Association: Diagnostic and Statistical Manual of Mental Disorders, 4th Edition. Washington, DC, American Psychiatric Association, 1994

Antelman SM: Time dependent sensitization as the cornerstone for a new approach to pharmacotherapy: drugs as foreign or stressful stimuli. Drug Dev Res 14:1–30, 1988

Arora FC, Fichtner CG, O'Connor F, et al: Paroxetine binding in the blood platelets of posttraumatic stress disorder patients. Life Sci 53:919–928, 1993

Baker DG, Diamond BI, Gilette G, et al: A double-blind, randomized, placebo-controlled, multicenter study of brofaromine in the treatment of posttraumatic stress disorder. Psychopharmacology (Berl) 122:386–389, 1995

Ballenger JC, Davidson JRT, Lecrubier Y, et al: Consensus statement on posttraumatic stress disorder from the International Consensus Group on Depression and Anxiety. J Clin Psychiatry 61(suppl 5):60–66, 2000

Bernstein GA, Garfinkel BD, Borchardt CM: Comparative studies of pharmacotherapy for school refusal. J Am Acad Child Adolesc Psychiatry 29:773–781, 1990

Bernstein GA, Anderson LK, Hektner JM, et al: Imipramine compliance in adolescents. J Am Acad Child Adolesc Psychiatry 39:284–291, 2000

Black B, Robbins DR: Panic disorder in children and adolescents. J Am Acad Child Adolesc Psychiatry 29:36–44, 1990

Blank A: The longitudinal course of posttraumatic stress disorder, in Posttraumatic Stress Disorder: DSM-IV and Beyond. Edited by Davidson J, Foa EB. Washington, DC, American Psychiatric Press, 1993, pp 3–22

Boscarino JA, Chang J: Electrocardiogram abnormalities among men with stress-related psychiatric disorders: implications for coronary artery disease and clinical research. Ann Behav Med 21:227–234, 1999

Bradburn IS: After the earth shook: children's stress symptoms 6–8 months after a disaster. Adv Behav Res Ther 13:173–179, 1991

Brady KT: Posttraumatic stress disorder and comorbidity: recognizing the many faces of PTSD. J Clin Psychiatry 58(suppl):12–15, 1997

Brady K, Pearlstein T, Asnis GM, et al: Efficacy and safety of sertraline treatment of posttraumatic stress disorder: a randomized controlled trial. JAMA 283:1837–1844, 2000

Brannon N, Labbate L, Huber M: Gabapentin treatment for posttraumatic stress disorder. Can J Psychiatry 45:84, 2000

Braun P, Greenberg D, Dasberg H, et al: Core symptoms of posttraumatic stress disorder unimproved by alprazolam treatment. J Clin Psychiatry 51:236–238, 1990

Bremner JD, Davis M, Southwick SM, et al: Neurobiology of posttraumatic stress disorder, in Review of Psychiatry, Vol 12. Edited by Oldham JM, Riba MB, Tasman A. Washington, DC, American Psychiatric Press, 1993, pp 183–205

Breslau N, Davis GC, Andreski P, et al: Traumatic events and posttraumatic stress disorder in an urban population of young adults. Arch Gen Psychiatry 48:216–222, 1991

Breslau N, Davis GC, Andreski P, et al: Sex differences in posttraumatic stress disorder. Arch Gen Psychiatry 54:1044–1048, 1997

Breslau N, Kessler RC, Chilcoat HD, et al: Trauma and posttraumatic stress disorder in the community: the 1996 Detroit Area Survey of Trauma. Arch Gen Psychiatry 55:626–632, 1998

Cahil L, Prims B, Weber M, et al: β-Adrenergic activation and memory for emotional events. Nature 371:702–704, 1994

Charney DS, Deutsch AY, Krystal JH, et al: Psychobiological mechanisms of posttraumatic stress disorder. Arch Gen Psychiatry 50:294–305, 1993

Connor KM, Sutherland SM, Tupler LA, et al: Fluoxetine in post-traumatic stress disorder: randomized, double-blind study. Br J Psychiatry 175:17–22, 1999

Cuffe SP, Addy CL, Garrison CZ, et al: Prevalence of PTSD in a community sample of older adolescents. J Am Acad Child Adolesc Psychiatry 37:147–154, 1998

Davidson JR: Pharmacotherapy of posttraumatic stress disorder: treatment options, long-term predictors of outcome. J Clin Psychiatry 61(suppl 5):52–56, 2000

Davidson J, Kudler H, Smith E, et al: Treatment of posttraumatic stress disorder with amitriptyline and placebo. Arch Gen Psychiatry 47:259–266, 1990

Davidson JRT, Kudler HS, Saunders WB, et al: Predicting response to amitriptyline in posttraumatic stress disorder. Am J Psychiatry 150: 1024–1029, 1993

Davidson JRT, Weisler RH, Malik ML, et al: Treatment of posttraumatic stress disorder with nefazodone. Int Clin Psychopharmacol 13:111–113, 1998

Davis L, Nugent A, Murray J, et al: Nefazodone treatment for chronic PTSD: an open trial (abstract). Biol Psychiatry 43:57S, 1998

De Bellis MD, Chrousos GP, Dorn LD, et al: H-P-A axis dysregulation in sexually abused girls. J Clin Endocrinol Metab 78:249–255, 1994

De Bellis MD, Baum AS, Birmaher B, et al: A.E. Bennett Research Award. Developmental traumatology, part I: biological stress systems. Biol Psychiatry 45:1259–1270, 1999a

De Bellis MD, Keshavan MS, Clark DB, et al: A.E. Bennett Research Award. Developmental traumatology, part II: brain development. Biol Psychiatry 45:1271–1284, 1999b

De Bellis MD, Keshavan MS, Spencer S, et al: N-Acetylaspartate concentration in the anterior cingulate of maltreated children and adolescents with PTSD. Am J Psychiatry 157:1175–1177, 2000

Deykin EY, Buka SL: Prevalence and risk factors for posttraumatic stress disorder among chemically dependent adolescents. Am J Psychiatry 154:752–757, 1997

Dillard ML, Bendfeldt F, Jernigan P: Use of thioridazine in post-traumatic stress disorder. South Med J 86:1276–1278, 1993

Domon SE, Andersen MS: Nefazodone for PTSD (letter). J Am Acad Child Adolesc Psychiatry 39:942–943, 2000

Donnelly CL, Amaya-Jackson L, March JS: Psychopharmacology of pediatric posttraumatic stress disorder. J Child Adolesc Psychopharmacol 9:203–220, 1999

Dow B, Kline N: Antidepressant treatment of posttraumatic stress disorder and major depression in veterans. Ann Clin Psychiatry 9:1–5, 1997

Famularo R, Kinscheiff R, Fenton T: Propranolol treatment for childhood posttraumatic stress disorder, acute type: a pilot study. Am J Dis Child 142:1244–1247, 1988

Famularo R, Kinscheiff R, Fenton T: Psychiatric diagnoses of maltreated children: preliminary findings. J Am Acad Child Adolesc Psychiatry 31:863–867, 1992

Famularo R, Fenton T, Augustyn M, et al: Persistence of pediatric post traumatic stress disorder after 2 years. Child Abuse and Neglect 20: 1245–1248, 1996

Feeney DJ, Klykylo W: Risperidone and tardive dyskinesia (letter). J Am Acad Child Adolesc Psychiatry 36:867, 1996

Fesler FA: Valproate in combat-related posttraumatic stress disorder. J Clin Psychiatry 52:361–364, 1991

Forster PL, Schoenfield FB, Marmar CR, et al: Lithium for irritability in post-traumatic stress disorder. J Trauma Stress 8:143–149, 1995

Foy DW, Madvig BT, Pynoos RS, et al: Etiologic factors in the development of posttraumatic stress disorder in children and adolescents. J School Psychol 34:133–145, 1996

Frederick CJ: Children traumatized by catastrophic situations, in Post-Traumatic Stress Disorder in Children. Edited by Eth S, Pynoos RS. Washington, DC, American Psychiatric Press, 1985, pp 71–100

Friedman MJ, Southwick SM: Towards pharmacotherapy for post-traumatic stress disorder, in Neurobiological and Clinical Consequences of Stress: From Normal Adaptation to PTSD. Edited by Friedman MJ, Charney DS, Deutsch AY. Philadelphia, PA, Lippincott-Raven, 1995, pp 465–481

Garland EJ, Smith DH: Case study: panic disorder on a child psychiatric consultation service. J Am Acad Child Adolesc Psychiatry 29:785–788, 1990

Garrison CZ, Bryant ES, Addy CL, et al: Posttraumatic stress disorder in adolescents after Hurricane Andrew. J Am Acad Child Adolesc Psychiatry 34:1193–1201, 1995

Gelpin E, Bonne O, Peri T, et al: Treatment of recent trauma survivors with benzodiazepines: a prospective study. J Clin Psychiatry 57:390–394, 1996

Giaconia RM, Reinherz HZ, Silverman AB, et al: Traumas and post-traumatic stress disorder in a community population of older adolescents. J Am Acad Child Adolesc Psychiatry 34:1369–1380, 1995

Gillette DW, Tannery LP: Beta-blocker inhibits tricyclic metabolism. J Am Acad Child Adolesc Psychiatry 33:223–224, 1994

Gittelman-Klein R, Klein DF: Controlled imipramine treatment of school phobia. Arch Gen Psychiatry 25:204–207, 1971

Glover H: A preliminary trial of nalmefene for the treatment of emotional numbing in combat veterans with post-traumatic stress disorder. Journal of Psychiatry and Related Sciences 30:225–263, 1993

Goenjian AK, Pynoos RS, Steinberg AM, et al: Psychiatric comorbidity in children after the 1988 earthquake in Armenia. J Am Acad Child Adolesc Psychiatry 34:1174–1184, 1995

Goenjian AK, Yehuda R, Pynoos RS, et al: Basal cortisol and dexamethasone suppression of cortisol among adolescents after the 1988 earthquake in Armenia. Am J Psychiatry 153:929–934, 1996

Green AH: Children traumatized by physical abuse, in Post-Traumatic Stress Disorder in Children. Edited by Eth S, Pynoos RS. Washington, DC, American Psychiatric Press, 1985, 133–154

Gupta S, Popli A, Bathurst E, et al: Efficacy of cyproheptadine for nightmares associated with posttraumatic stress disorder. Compr Psychiatry 39:160–164, 1998

Guy W (ed): ECDEU Assessment Manual for Psychopharmacology, Revised. U.S. Department of Health, Education, and Welfare publication (ADM) no. 76-338. Rockville, MD, National Institute of Mental Health, 1976

Hamner M, Ulmer H, Horne D: Buspirone potentiation of antidepressants in the treatment of PTSD. Depression and Anxiety 5:137–139, 1997

Hamner MB, Loberbaum JP, George MS: Potential role of the anterior cingulate cortex in PTSD: review and hypothesis. Depression and Anxiety 9:1–14, 1999

Harmon RJ, Riggs PD: Clonidine for posttraumatic stress disorder in preschool children. J Am Acad Child Adolesc Psychiatry 35:1247–1249, 1996

Heim C, Newport J, Heit S, et al: Pituitary-adrenal and autonomic responses to stress in women after sexual and physical abuse in childhood. JAMA 284:592–597, 2000

Hertzberg MA, Feldman ME, Beckham JC, et al: Trial of trazodone for posttraumatic stress disorder using a multiple baseline group design. J Clin Psychopharmacol 16:294–298, 1996

Hertzberg MA, Butterfield MI, Feldman ME, et al: A preliminary study of lamotrigine for the treatment of posttraumatic stress disorder. Biol Psychiatry 45:1226–1229, 1999

Hidalgo R, Hertzberg MA, Mellman T, et al: Nefazadone in post-traumatic stress disorder: results from six open-label trials. Int Clin Psychopharmacol 14:61–68, 1999

Holsboer F, van Bardelen U, Gerken A, et al: Blunted corticotrophin and normal cortisol responses to human corticotrophin-releasing factor in depression. N Engl J Med 311:1127, 1984

Horrigan JP: Risperidone appears effective for children, adolescents with severe PTSD. Presented at the American Academy of Child and Adolescent Psychiatry meeting, Anaheim, CA, October 1998

Horrigan JP, Barnhill LJ: The supression of nightmares with guanfacine. J Clin Psychiatry 57:371, 1996

Hubbard J, Realmuto GM, Northwood AK, et al: Comorbidity of psychiatric diagnosis with posttraumatic stress disorder. J Am Acad Child Adolesc Psychiatry 34:1167–1173, 1995

Kessler RC, Sonnega A, Bromet E, et al: Posttraumatic stress disorder in the National Comorbidity Survey. Arch Gen Psychiatry 52:1048–1060, 1995

Kinzie JD, Leung P: Clonidine in Cambodian patients with post-traumatic stress disorder. J Nerv Ment Dis 177:546–550, 1989

Kitchner I, Greenstein R: Low dose lithium carbonate in the treatment of post-traumatic stress disorder: brief communication. Military Medicine 150:378–381, 1985

Kolb LC, Burris BC, Griffiths S: Propranolol and clonidine in treatment of the chronic posttraumatic stress disorders of war, in Post-Traumatic Stress Disorder: Psychological and Biological Sequelae. Edited by van der Kolk BA. Washington, DC, American Psychiatric Press, 1984

Kosten TR, Frank JB, Dan E, et al: Pharmacotherapy for posttraumatic stress disorder using phenelzine or imipramine. J Nerv Ment Dis 179:366–370, 1991

Krashin D, Oates EW: Risperidone as an adjunct therapy for post-traumatic stress disorder. Military Medicine 164:605–606, 1999

Kutcher SP, Reiter S, Gardner DM, et al: The pharmacotherapy of anxiety disorders in children and adolescents. Psychiatr Clin North Am 15:41–67, 1992

LaPorta JD, Ware MR: Buspirone and the treatment of posttraumatic stress disorder. J Clin Psychopharmacol 12:133–134, 1992

Le Doux JE : The Emotional Brain: The Mysterious Underpinnings of Emotional Life. New York, Simon and Schuster, 1996

Leonard HL, March J, Rickler KC, et al: Pharmacology of the selective serotonin reuptake inhibitors in children and adolescents. J Am Acad Child Adolesc Psychiatry 36:725–736, 1997

Leyba CM, Wampler TP: Risperidone in PTSD. Psychiatr Serv 49:245–246, 1998

Lipper S, Davidson JRT, Grady TA, et al: Preliminary study of carbamazepine in posttraumatic stress disorder. Psychosomatics 27:849–854, 1986

Looff D, Grimley P, Kuiler F, et al: Carbamazepine for posttraumatic stress disorder (letter). J Am Acad Child Adolesc Psychiatry 34:703–704, 1995

Lowenstein RJ, Hornstein N, Farber B: Open trial of clonazepam in the treatment of post-traumatic stress symptoms in multiple personality disorder. Dissociation 1:3–12, 1988

March JS, Amaya-Jackson L, Pynoos RS: Pediatric posttraumatic stress disorder, in Textbook of Child and Adolescent Psychiatry, 2nd Edition. Edited by Weiner JM. Washington, DC, American Psychiatric Press, 1996

March J, Cohen J, Berliner L: Treatment of children and adolescents, in Effective Treatments for PTSD: Practice Guidelines from the International Society for Traumatic Stress Studies. Edited by Foa EB, Keane TM, Friedman MJ. New York, Guilford, 2000

Marmar CK, Foy D, Kagan B, et al: An integrated approach for treating posttraumatic stress, in Posttraumatic Stress Disorder: A Clinical Review. Edited by Pynoos RS. Lutherville, MD, Sidran Press, 1993

Marmar CR, Schoenfeld F, Weiss DS: Open trial of fluvoxamine treatment for combat-related posttraumatic stress disorder. J Clin Psychiatry 14:79–81, 1996

Marshall RD, Schneier FR, Fallon BA, et al: An open trial of paroxetine in patients with noncombat-related, chronic posttraumatic stress disorder. J Clin Psychopharmacol 18:10–18, 1998

Mazza JJ: The relationship between posttraumatic stress symptomatology and suicidal behavior in school-based adolescents. Suicide Life Threat Behav 30:91–103, 2000

McCloskey LA, Walker M: Posttraumatic stress in children exposed to family violence and single-event trauma. J Am Acad Child Adolesc Psychiatry 39:108–115, 2000

McFarlane AC: Posttraumatic stress disorder: a model of the longitudinal course and the role of risk factors. J Clin Psychiatry 61(suppl):15–20, 2000

Monnelly EP, Ciraulo DA: Risperidone effects on irritable aggression in posttraumatic stress disorder. J Clin Psychopharmacol 19:377–378, 1999

Nader K, Pynoos R, Fairbanks L, et al: Children's PTSD reactions one year after a sniper attack at their school. Am J Psychiatry 147:1526–1530, 1990

Nader KO, Pynoos RS, Fairbanks LA, et al: A preliminary study of PTSD and grief among children of Kuwait following the Gulf crisis. Br J Clin Psychol 32:407–416, 1993

Nader K, Blake D, Kriegler J, et al: Clinician-Administered PTSD Scale for Children (CAPS-C), Current and Lifetime Diagnosis Version, and Instruction Manual. Los Angeles, CA, UCLA Neuropsychiatric Institute and National Center for PTSD, 1994

Neal LA, Shapland W, Fox C: An open trial of moclobemide in the treatment of posttraumatic stress disorder. Int Clin Psychopharmacol 12:231–237, 1997

Nutt DJ: The psychobiology of posttraumatic stress disorder. J Clin Psychiatry 61(suppl): 24–29, 2000

Penava SJ, Otto MW, Pollack MH, et al: Current status of pharmacotherapy for PTSD: an effect size analysis of controlled studies. Depression and Anxiety 4:240–242, 1997

Perkonigg A, Kessler RC, Storz S, et al: Traumatic events and post-traumatic stress disorder in the community: prevalence and comorbidity. Acta Psychiatr Scand 101:46–59, 2000

Perrin S, Smith P, Yule W: The assessment and treatment of post-traumatic stress disorder in children and adolescents. J Child Psychol Psychiatry 41:277–289, 2000

Perry BD: Neurobiological sequelae of childhood trauma: PTSD in children, in Catecholamine Function in Post-Traumatic Stress Disorder: Emerging Concepts. Edited by Murburg MM. Washington, DC, American Psychiatric Press, 1994, pp 233–255

Pfefferbaum B: Posttraumatic stress disorder in children: a review of the past 10 years. J Am Acad Child Adolesc Psychiatry 36:1503–1511, 1997

Post RM, Kopanda RT: Cocaine, kindling, and psychosis. Am J Psychiatry 133:627–634, 1976

Preskorn SH, Alderman J, Chung M, et al: Pharmacokinetics of desipramine coadministered with sertraline or fluoxetine. J Clin Psychopharmacol 14:90–98, 1994

Pynoos RS, Frederick CJ, Nader K, et al: Life threat and posttraumatic stress disorder in school-age children. Arch Gen Psychiatry 44:1057–1063, 1987

Risse SC, Whitters A, Burke J, et al: Severe withdrawal symptoms after discontinuation of alprazolam in eight patients with combat-induced posttraumatic stress disorder. J Clin Psychiatry 51:206–209, 1990

Robert R, Blakeney PE, Villareal C, et al: Imipramine treatment in pediatric burn patients with symptoms of acute stress disorder: a pilot study. J Am Acad Child Adolesc Psychiatry 38:873–882, 1999

Schwab-Stone M, Chen C, Greenberger E, et al: No safe haven II: the effects of violence exposure on urban youth. J Am Acad Child Adolesc Psychiatry 38:359–367, 1999

Seedat S, Lockhat R, Kaminer D, et al: An open trial of citalopram in adolescents with post-traumatic stress disorder. Int Clin Psychopharmacol, in press

Shalev A, Bleich A, Ursano RJ: Posttraumatic stress disorder: somatic comorbidity and effort tolerance. Psychosomatics 31:197–203, 1990

Shaw JA, Applegate B, Tanner S, et al: Psychological effects of Hurricane Andrew on an elementary school population. J Am Acad Child Adolesc Psychiatry 34:1185–1192, 1995

Silva RR, Alpert M, Munoz DM, et al: Stress and vulnerability to posttraumatic stress disorder in children and adolescents. Am J Psychiatry 157:1229–1235, 2000

Southwick SM, Krystal JH, Bremner JD: Noradrenergic and serotonergic function in posttraumatic stress disorder. Arch Gen Psychiatry 54:749–758, 1997

Stein MB, Koverola C, Hanna C, et al: Hippocampal volume in women victimized by childhood sexual abuse. Psychol Med 27:951–959, 1997

Terr LC: Childhood traumas: an outline and overview. Am J Psychiatry 148:10–20, 1991

Tucker P, Smith KL, Marx B, et al: Fluvoxamine reduces physiologic reactivity to trauma scripts in posttraumatic stress disorder. J Clin Psychopharmacol 20:367–372, 2000

van der Kolk BA, Greenberg MS, Orr SP: Endogenous opioids, stress induced analgesia and posttraumatic stress disorder. Psychopharmacol Bull 25: 417–421, 1989

van der Kolk BA, Dreyfuss D, Michaels M, et al: Fluoxetine in posttraumatic stress disorder. J Clin Psychiatry 55:517–522, 1994

Vrana S, Lauterbach D: Prevalence of traumatic events and posttraumatic psychological symptoms in a nonclinical sample of college students. J Trauma Stress 7:289–302, 1994

Weisenberg M, Schwarzwald J, Waysman M, et al: Coping of school-age children in the sealed room during scud missile bombardment and postwar stress reactions. J Consult Clin Psychol 61:462–467, 1993

Wells BG, Chu CC, Johnson E, et al: Buspirone in the treatment of posttraumatic stress disorder. Pharmacotherapy 11:340–343, 1991

Yehuda R: Recent developments in the neuroendocrinology of posttraumatic stress disorder. CNS Spectrums 3(suppl):23–29, 1998

Yehuda R, McFarlane AC: Conflict between current knowledge about posttraumatic stress disorder and its original conceptual basis. Am J Psychiatry 152:1705–1713, 1995

Yehuda R, Southwick SM, Krystal JM, et al: Enhanced suppression of cortisol following dexamethasone administration in combat veterans with and without posttraumatic stress disorder. Am J Psychiatry 150:83–86, 1993

Yehuda R, Boisoneau D, Lowy MT, et al: Dose-response changes in plasma cortisol and lymphocyte glucocorticoid receptors following dexamethasone administration in combat veterans with and without posttraumatic stress disorder. Arch Gen Psychiatry 52:583–593, 1995

Yehuda R, Levengood R, Schmeidler J, et al: Increased pituitary activation following metyrapone administration in PTSD. Psychoneuroendocrinology 21:1–16, 1996

Yehuda R, Bierer LM, Schmeidler J, et al: Low cortisol and risk for PTSD in adult offspring of Holocaust survivors. Am J Psychiatry 157:1252–1259, 2000

Chapter 5

Relationship Between Childhood Traumatic Experiences and PTSD in Adults

Rachel Yehuda, Ph.D.
Ilyse L. Spertus, Ph.D.
Julia A. Golier, M.D.

Introduction

There has been a burgeoning interest in examining the impact of childhood trauma on the mental and physical health of the adult. This chapter seeks primarily to review evidence for the association between early traumatic life events, particularly a history of repeated physical or sexual abuse, and the subsequent development of posttraumatic stress disorder (PTSD) in adulthood. This relationship will be considered in the context of theory and data on the impact of early stress on developing neurobiologic systems. One of the most pivotal observations in relation to the development of PTSD in adults traumatized as children has been the association between early trauma exposure and subsequent retraumatization. This chapter considers the possibility that changes in neurobiologic systems resulting from adverse childhood experiences can result in augmented responses to subsequent stressors experienced in adulthood. These augmented responses render survivors more vulnerable to the development

This work was supported by NIMH 49555 (RY). We would like to thank Eyal Shemesh, M.D., for his thoughtful suggestions.

of PTSD and related problems. To provide necessary perspectives about conclusions in the literature and highlight gaps in our knowledge, we also consider methodologic issues related to the study of the impact early events have on subsequent symptoms.

Long-Term Consequences of Childhood Maltreatment—Sexual Abuse, Physical Abuse, Emotional Abuse, and/or Neglect

One of the cornerstones of current biopsychosocial formulations of psychopathology is that negative life events, particularly those that occur early in development, play a major etiologic role in precipitating and/or exacerbating psychologic disorder in adults. This idea has been empirically validated by studies demonstrating strong associations between the experience of early childhood trauma and subsequent psychologic problems in adulthood (see Table 5–1; see also reviews by Beitchman et al. 1992; Briere and Elliot 1994; Briere and Runtz 1991; Browne and Finkelhor 1986; Cahill et al. 1991; Cloitre et al. 1996; A.H. Green 1993; Kendall-Tackett et al. 1993; Malinsky-Rummell and Hansen 1993; Mullen et al. 1996; Weiss et al. 1999).

Symptoms of PTSD are prominent among the mental health problems that can be present in adults who report childhood maltreatment (Bremner et al. 1993; Briggs and Joyce 1997; Cloitre et al. 1997; Ellason et al. 1996; Elliot and Briere 1995; Epstein et al. 1997, 1998; Follette et al. 1994; Gelinas 1983; Lawrence et al. 1995; Lindberg and Distad 1985; McNew and Abell 1995; Rodriguez et al. 1996, 1997; Roesler and McKenzie 1994; Schaaf and McCanne 1998; Silverman et al. 1996; Triffleman et al. 1995; Widom 1999; Wind and Silvern 1994; Zlotnick 1997; Zlotnick et al. 1996). However, most observations regarding the relationship between early experiences and adult PTSD have been retrospective and have relied on examination of clinical populations. Nonetheless, investigators have successfully linked adult PTSD symptoms to aspects of early trauma exposure (e.g., degree of life threat, physical injury, testifying about rape, penetration) (Epstein et al. 1997). These observations imply that the impact of early maltreatment on PTSD symptoms can be long lasting.

Many psychologic problems have been documented in adults maltreated as children, and some appear to be at least as prominent as PTSD. Other mental health consequences in the adult related to early sexual and/or physical trauma include anxiety (Briere and Runtz 1988; Briere et al. 1988; Bushnell et al. 1992; Collings 1995; Elliot and Briere 1995; Fromuth 1986; Gorcey et al. 1986; Greenwald et al. 1990; Herman and Schatzow 1987; Mancini et al. 1995; McCauley et al. 1997; McNew and Abell 1995; Moeller et al. 1993; Sedney and Brooks 1984; Wenninger and Ehlers 1998; Zlotnick et al. 1996), depression (Boudewyn and Liem 1995; Briere and Runtz 1988; Briere et al. 1988, 1997; Bushnell et al. 1992; Cloitre et al. 1997; Collings 1995; Ellason et al. 1996; Elliot and Briere 1995; Fromuth and Burkhart 1989; Luntz and Widom 1994; Mancini et al. 1995; McCauley et al. 1997; Moeller et al. 1993; Mullen et al. 1996; DePaul and Domenech 2000; Peters 1988; Roesler and McKenzie 1994; Sedney and Brooks 1984; Silverman et al. 1996; J.A. Stein et al. 1988; Wenninger and Ehlers 1998; Wind and Silvern 1994), suicidality (Bagley and Ramsey 1986; Boudewyn and Liem 1995; Briere and Runtz 1987; Briere et al. 1988, 1997; G.R. Brown and Anderson 1991; Bryer et al. 1987; Cloitre et al. 1997; McCauley et al. 1997; Silverman et al. 1996; van der Kolk et al. 1991), dissociation (Briere and Runtz 1987; Briere et al. 1988, 1997; Chu and Dill 1990; Cloitre et al. 1997; Dancu et al. 1996; Ellason et al. 1996; Elliot and Briere 1995; Gelinas 1983; Lawrence et al. 1995; Nash et al. 1993; Roesler and McKenzie 1994; Wenninger and Ehlers 1998; Zlotnick 1997; Zlotnick et al. 1996), personality disorders (G.R. Brown and Anderson 1991; Johnson et al. 2000; Luntz and Widom 1994; Raczek 1992; Silverman et al. 1996), and substance abuse (Briere et al. 1988, 1997; G.R. Brown and Anderson 1991; Bushnell et al. 1992; Ellason et al. 1996; Epstein et al. 1998; Fleming et al. 1999; Kunitz et al. 1998; Luntz and Widom 1994; McCauley et al. 1997; Merrill et al. 1999; Moeller et al. 1993; Mullen et al. 1996; Silverman et al. 1996; Swett et al. 1991; Triffleman et al. 1995).

More general problems, particularly among those who experienced sexual abuse, include impaired sexual functioning (Brunngraber 1986; Finkelhor 1979; Gold 1986; Herman 1981; Lindberg and Distad 1985; Meiselman 1978; J.A. Stein et al. 1988; Tsai et al.

Table 5–1. Studies examining the relationship between childhood

Citations	Popu-lation[1]	Sample size, n (abused)[2]	Gender	Type of study[3]	Type of trauma[4]
Sedney and Brooks 1984	CS	301 (NR)	Females	R	SA
Lindberg and Distad 1985	PO	17 (17)	Females	R	SA
Briere and Runtz 1988	CS	251 (NR)	Females	R	PA,E
Briere 1988	PO	195 (133)	Females	R	SA
Briere et al. 1988	PO	80 (40)	Both	R	SA
Harter and Alexander 1988	CS	85 (29)	Females	R	SA
Fromuth and Burkhart 1989	CS	582 (NR)	Males	R	SA
Chu and Dill 1990	PI	98 (62)	Females	R	SA,PA
Greenwald et al. 1990	HCP	108 (54)	Females	R	SA
Brown and Anderson 1991	PI	947 (166)	Both	R	SA,PA
van der Kolk et al. 1991	C, PO, CJ	74 (NR)	Both	R	SA, PA, N,W
Bushnell et al. 1992	C	301 (NR)	Females	R	SA
Bremner et al. 1993	PO, MS	66 (NR)	Males	R	PA
Moeller et al. 1993	MS	668 (354)	Females	R	SA, PA, E
Nash et al. 1993	PO, C	105 (56)	Females	R	SA
Follette et al. 1994	C, HCP	558 (NR)	Both	R	SA
Roesler and McKenzie 1994	PO	188 (188)	Both	R	SA
Wind and Silvern 1994	C	259 (41)	Females	R	SA,PA
Boudewyn and Liem 1995	CS	438 (91)	Both	R	SA
Collings 1995	CS	284 (82)	Males	R	SA
Elliot and Briere 1995	C	505 (116)	Both	R	SA
Mancini et al. 1995	PO	205 (104)	Both	R	SA, PA
McNew and Abell 1995	PO	127 (70)	Both	R	SA
Triffleman et al. 1995	PI	46 (34)	Males	R	SA,PA,N,W, S
Dancu et al. 1996	AT	158 (41)	Females	R	SA
Ellason et al. 1996	PI	106 (69)	Both	R	SA,PA
Lawrence et al. 1995	PO	46 (46)	Females	R	SA
Mullen et al. 1996	C	497 (107)	Females	R	SA,PA,E
Rodriguez et al. 1996	PO	117 (117)	Both	R	SA
Silverman et al. 1996	C	375 (40)	Both	P	SA,PA
Zlotnick et al. 1996	PI	108 (74)	Females	R	SA
Briere et al. 1997	PE	93 (44)	Females	R	SA,PA
Briggs and Joyce 1997	PO	73 (73)	Females	R	SA
Cloitre et al. 1997	C	56 (24)	Females	R	SA

maltreatment and psychologic symptoms in adults

Familial environment controlled[5]	PTSD	Anxiety	Depression	Suicidal ideation/ suicide attempts	Disso- ciation	Sub- stance abuse	Revictimization in adulthood
		X	X				
	X						
		X	X	X	X		
				X	X	X	X
		X	X	X	X		X
X							
			X				
					X		
X		X					
				X		X	
				X			
		X	X			X	
	X						
		X		X		X	X
X					X		
	X						
	X		X		X		
X	X		X				X
			X	X			X
X		X	X				
	X	X	X		X		
		X	X				
	X	X					
	X					X	
					X		
	X		X		X	X	
	X				X		
X			X	X		X	
	X						
	X		X	X		X	
	X	X			X		X
			X	X		X	X
	X						
	X		X	X	X		X

Table 5–2. Studies examining the relationship between childhood

Citations	Popu-lation[1]	Sample size, n (abused)[2]	Gender	Type of study[3]	Type of trauma[4]
Epstein et al. 1997	C	3220 (288)	Females	R	SA
McCauley et al. 1997	MS	1931 (424)	Females	R	SA,PA
Rodriguez et al. 1997	PO	76 (45)	Females	R	SA
Roth et al. 1997	PO, C	234 (113)	Both	R	SA,PA
Styron and Janoff-Bulman 1997	CS	879 (232)	Both	R	SA,PA,E
Zlotnick 1997	CJ	85 (56)	Females	R	SA,PA
Epstein et al. 1998	C	2994 (281)	Females	R	SA
Kunitz et al. 1998	PO, C	734 (NR)	Both	R	SA,PA
Schaaf and McCanne 1998	CS	322 (111)	Females	R	SA,PA
Wenninger and Ehlers (study 1) 1998	C	72 (43)	Females	R	SA
Wenninger and Ehlers (study 2) 1998	C	35 (35)	Females	R	SA
Fleming et al. 1999	C	710 (144)	Females	R	SA
Merrill et al. 1999	C	1093 (NR)	Females	R	SA,PA
Widom 1999	CJ	1196 (676)	Both	P	SA,PA,N
Nishith et al. 2000	AT	117 (117)	Females	R	SA
DePaul and Domenech 2000	MS	48 (NR)	Females	R	PA,E

[1]Sample used in the study.
AT = adult trauma; C = community; CJ = criminal justice system; CS = college students; CT = child trauma follow-up as adults; HCP= health care professionals; PE= psychiatry emergency room; PI = psychiatry inpatient; PO= psychiatry outpatient.
[2]*n* represents the total number of participants used in these analyses to determine the relationship between childhood maltreatment and psychologic symptoms in adulthood. The number in parentheses reflects the number of participants in each study that reported childhood maltreatment. NR=not reported in this format.
[3]P=prospective; R=retrospective.

Familial environment controlled[6]	PTSD	Anxiety	Depression	Suicidal ideation/ suicide attempts	Disso- ciation	Sub- stance abuse	Revictimization in adulthood
	X						
		X	X	X		X	
	X						
	X						
X			X				
	X				X		
	X					X	
						X	X
	X						X
		X	X		X		
		X	X				
X						X	X
						X	X
X	X						X
							X
			X				X[6]

[4]E=emotional abuse; N=neglect; PA=physical abuse; S=separation; SA=sexual abuse; W=witnessed trauma.

[5]Studies that included the effects of childhood familial environment in their analyses when studying the relationship between childhood maltreatment and adult psychopathology.

[6]In this case, authors examined participants' potential for perpetration of childhood abuse rather than revictimization.

1979), interpersonal problems (Kendall-Tackett and Simon 1988; Wyatt and Newcomb 1990), and physical illness (Felitti 1991). The myriad outcomes associated with physical or sexual trauma in childhood warrant the conclusion that there are no certain or simple outcomes associated with childhood trauma exposure.

Challenges in Formulating a Model of the Effects of Early Child Maltreatment on the Adult

The wide range and lack of specificity of negative outcomes associated with early trauma present a challenge to formulating a cohesive model for the effects of early trauma on the adult. Indeed, although numerous outcomes have been identified as occurring more often in adults who were traumatized as children than in those who were not, no single outcome has been shown to be a specific indicator of early trauma. Furthermore, the outcomes that have been identified as occurring more often in adult survivors of childhood trauma can also occur in adults traumatized in adulthood and in the absence of traumatic experiences. Given the prevalence of early trauma, particularly in treatment-seeking populations, clinicians are increasingly focused on considering the extent to which these early traumatic experiences are relevant to patients' current symptoms and whether and how these experiences should be addressed in therapy. However, at this stage, there are no definitive behavioral markers of childhood maltreatment that could aid in the clinical assessment of such patients.

It is important to note that the above summary of the enduring effects of trauma applies to the literature on child maltreatment as a whole rather than to specific effects that may result from specific types of events or combinations of events. Such analyses may ultimately reveal more explicit patterns of outcome related to particular lifetime events or the cumulative effects of stress. To date, most studies have examined the impact of childhood sexual and physical abuse. These events, by nature, are usually chronic and repeated rather than single-episode occurrences and also occur in the context of other negative life events and circumstances (i.e., neglect, complex familial and interpersonal dynamics, sociodemographic and economic considerations). These circumstances may also contribute to psychopathology, but their effects have not systematically been considered in studies examining the impact of sexual or physical abuse per se.

Because PTSD is thought to also occur after single-episode events (DSM-IV; American Psychiatric Association 1994), it is important to examine the long-term impact of these events as well, such as random shootings in schools or other public places; terrorism; accidents and natural disasters; single episodes of assault; and life-threatening illnesses. These studies will be critical in sorting out the consequences related to the nature of exposure from those related to other risk factors associated with chronic traumatization. Unfortunately, there is a paucity of information on the long-term outcome of such events and no studies whatsoever examining the long-term neurobiologic consequences of such experiences in the adult. Evaluating the long-term consequences of such events requires the passage of time, and few investigators were interested in the long-term effects of single-episode events before the diagnosis of PTSD was established. Such studies will invariably appear, however, and it will be critical to examine whether single-episode events are associated with a set of psychologic, social, physical, behavioral, and cognitive consequences that is similar to that of those related to more complex exposures such as physical and sexual abuse. Preliminary evidence from a small number of prospective and retrospective studies on the long-term effects of such events suggests that although the effects of such events may linger, they are not associated with the same degree of psychopathology seen in adults exposed to childhood maltreatment.

Long-Term Consequences of Single-Episode Traumatic Events: Preliminary Evidence

There have been some longitudinal studies of adults exposed to devastating disaster as children. The earliest study investigated psychiatric symptoms in survivors of the floods following the collapse of the Buffalo Creek dam in 1972. The collapse of the dam unleashed millions of gallons of sludge and water in a narrow valley, killing 125 residents. An original sample of 207 children was studied in 1974 (Gleser et al. 1981; Green et al. 1991). About half of the subjects were available for a follow-up 17 years later. The results of follow-up evaluations suggested that there had been substantial decreases in overall symptom severity ratings of anxiety, belligerence, somatic symptoms, and agitation. Only 7% of those studied met criteria for PTSD, compared with a postflood rate of 32%. All of the subjects with PTSD at follow-up were women. Of note was the observation that some symptoms, such as substance abuse and suicidal ideation, increased over time—that is, they were not present in the children but had emerged by the time of follow-up. Despite this, however, the results suggested that by adulthood there had been "recovery" from symptoms related to the floods, especially posttraumatic symptoms (Green et al. 1994).

The long-term impact of a terrorist attack in Israel was also investigated retrospectively in subjects who had survived the incident as children 17 years earlier (Desivilya et al. 1996). The incident took place in 1974 in the town of Ma'a lot. A group of 120 high school children was seized and taken hostage by armed Palestinian guerillas. During the 16-hour kidnapping, 22 adolescents were killed and many were severely wounded. Of the surviving victims, 59 were available for study and were assessed for mental health symptoms. About half of them reported having experienced five to eight of the 17 symptoms of PTSD in the month prior to the interview. They also reported having symptom exacerbations after hearing of current terrorist events that reminded them of their experiences, events that occur not infrequently in Israel. Insofar as adults who had been physically injured during the attack reported more mental health symptoms than those who had not been injured, the authors concluded that symptoms were related to objective characteristics of the trauma. In a similar study, Tyano et al. (1996) examined 389 subjects during compulsory army services who filled out questionnaires about a bus–train collision they had been involved with 7 years earlier. This retrospective study also demonstrated that subjects reporting a high degree of exposure were more likely to report relatively high levels of somatization, depression, phobic anxiety, psychoticism, and PTSD symptoms. These studies demonstrate that some individuals who survive a single-episode traumatic event in childhood report posttraumatic symptoms in adulthood, long after the event is over. However, the great majority of subjects show a decline in symptoms of PTSD and a complete recovery from this disorder. Furthermore, although symptoms are present in some survivors years after the event, the myriad problems that have been associated with sexual and/or physical abuse or neglect have not been observed following single-incident traumas.

The lack of prospective studies evaluating the long-term impact of such events reflects the fact that PTSD is a relatively new diagnosis. However, data regarding the long-term impact of single-episode events will be available in the near future. Indeed, prospective, longitudinal examinations on traumatized children are under way. These studies suggest that the recovery from single-episode events such as disasters may occur within a relatively short period of time. Winje and Ulvik (1998), who studied 28 Swedish children 1 and 3 years after a bus accident, demonstrated a marked reduction in PTSD symptoms at 3 years as compared with those at 1 year. Symptoms present in the children at 3-year follow-up correlated with their mothers' symptoms rather than with the nature of their traumatic exposure. Similarly, Israeli preschool children who had been exposed to SCUD missiles during the Persian Gulf War also showed substantial symptom improvement at a 30-month follow-up. Again, symptoms present in children at this time were correlated with levels of maternal avoidant symptoms (Laor et al. 1997), suggesting familial and/or environmental factors mediate posttraumatic symptoms following childhood trauma.

Prevalence of PTSD in Children and Adults Following Childhood Trauma

The literature examining rates of PTSD among children who have survived trauma does not present a uniform estimate of the prevalence of this condition. Not surprisingly, estimates of PTSD vary considerably depending on the type of event experienced, the population studied, and the sampling and diagnostic methods used. Generally speaking, rates of PTSD following extreme violence are quite high; for example, rates of PTSD after being kidnapped, witnessing the murder of a parent, or experiencing domestic violence situations have ranged from 95%–100% (Horowitz et al. 1995; Kinzie et al. 1986; Pynoos et al. 1987; Schwartz and Kowalski 1991; Terr 1981). The diagnoses of PTSD in children after such experiences are often made soon after the traumatic event. Studies examining children immediately after natural disasters have found PTSD to occur in anywhere from 3% to 87% of the children (Garrison et al. 1995; Shannon et al. 1994; Shaw et al. 1995). The prevalence of PTSD after sexual or physical abuse in children has been reported to be from 21% (Deblinger et al. 1989) to 48%–55% (Kiser et al. 1991). What appears to emerge is a pattern in which some types of events are associated with a high degree of recovery, whereas others are not. As noted, studies examining PTSD after exposure to natural disasters or accidents have almost unanimously shown that the rate of PTSD declines in children over time. Even exposure to extreme events such as war is associated with recovery in children (Sack et al. 1993).

Interestingly, the prevalence of PTSD in children reported for childhood sexual abuse appears to be lower than the prevalence of PTSD in adults traumatized in childhood. Indeed, most studies of adults who report abuse in childhood show a much higher range of PTSD, ranging from 72% to 100% (Lindberg and Distad 1985; Rodriguez et al. 1997). Although methodologic differences may explain some of the discrepancy, it is interesting to speculate about other explanations. The finding of a higher prevalence of PTSD in adults exposed to childhood physical or sexual abuse suggests that the full impact of early childhood abuse may not be realized until adulthood, particularly if no steps are taken to help the child overcome these experiences when he or she is young. Beitchman et al. (1992) referred to "sleeper" effects of abuse that require developmental maturity for their expression. Such effects are not evident as short-term consequences of a trauma but may emerge subsequently. An example of such an effect is sexual dysfunction, which has clearly been associated with childhood sexual abuse but may not be evident until adulthood.

The appearance of some psychologic responses to early trauma may require more developed cognition and maturity. As one's perspective and cognitive capacities develop with age, an adult's perceptions and responses to an earlier experience can change as well. Thus, it is possible for adults to have delayed reactions to earlier events as they become more fully aware of the magnitude of danger or betrayal implied by an experience. Furthermore, subsequent life circumstances can either confirm or negate cognitions associated with childhood trauma. That is, to the extent that children can be removed from a traumatic situation and placed in an environment in which they can thrive, they may be able to alter their perception about their personal safety. Accordingly, it is important to anticipate how early traumatic events may set the stage for a process that may require incubation, development, and modification by further environmental effects.

The failure to observe as high a rate of PTSD in children compared with adults who report having been sexually and physically abused as children also suggests the possibility that trauma symptoms are related not only to early experiences but to subsequent exposures as well. Following a natural disaster or random violence, a child may mobilize coping resources from family and other sources of social support, but following sexual or physical abuse such supports are seldom available. We suggest in the next section that one of the most devastating consequences of early maltreatment is the increased likelihood of further victimization. This phenomenon has not been observed or studied in children who have survived other types of adverse experiences.

Impact of Early Maltreatment on Reaction to Subsequent Trauma and Risk of Revictimization

The experience of childhood maltreatment appears to increase the likelihood of further victimization (Boudewyn and Liem 1995; Briere 1988; Briere et al. 1988, 1997; Cloitre et al. 1997; Fleming et al. 1999; Follette et al. 1996; Kunitz et al. 1998; Merrill et al. 1999; Moeller et al. 1993; Nishith et al. 2000; Schaaf and McCanne 1998; Widom 1999; Wind and Silvern 1994; Zlotnick et al. 1996).

Studies of adult sexual assault victims have documented a high degree of revictimization (Briere and Runtz 1987; Ellis et al. 1982; Gidycz et al. 1993; Koss and Dinero 1989; Marhoefer-Dvorak et al. 1988; Roth et al. 1990; Sorenson et al. 1991). Retrospective studies demonstrate a high rate of childhood sexual assault in rape survivors (Briere and Runtz 1988; Kendall-Tackett and Simon 1988; Russell 1986; Wyatt and Newcomb 1990). In fact, early childhood victimization is the single best predictor of subsequent victimization (Alexander and Lupfer 1987; Briere and Runtz 1987; Briere et al. 1997; Fromuth et al. 1986; Russell 1986) and, more importantly, of symptoms following subsequent victimization (Norris and Kaniasty 1994).

It has been demonstrated on the basis of retrospective studies that individuals who develop PTSD in response to events that occur in adulthood are more likely to have had earlier traumatic experiences, particularly childhood physical and sexual abuse (Bremner et al. 1993; Zlotnick 1997). However, to the extent that such subjects also have experienced trauma in adulthood, it is difficult to state with conviction that current PTSD symptoms are associated with past abuse experiences unless other important variables are taken into account. Rather, it appears that early maltreatment in combination with other individual characteristics and subsequent exposure variables may increase the risk for PTSD.

Indeed, strong support for the relationship between early abuse and subsequent victimization as the mediator of adult PTSD is provided by Widom's powerful prospective study of victims of substantiated child abuse and neglect who were followed until adulthood (Widom 1999). In the first phase of this research, children were identified through an examination of official criminal records containing reports of abuse or neglect between 1967 and 1971 in a Midwestern metropolitan county and compared with children who were matched for age, race, gender, and socioeconomic status. Twenty years after the abuse occurred, 83% of the original sample was tracked down and interviewed. The final report was based on diagnostic interviews of 676 abused and 520 comparison subjects. A prevalence rate of 20.4% of current or lifetime PTSD was found in the comparison subjects. The prevalence rates of PTSD were higher in those who had suffered abuse in childhood. Specifically, the rate was 37.5% in those who had experienced childhood sexual abuse, 32.7% in those who had experienced physical abuse, and 30.6% in those who had experienced neglect. The group that had been maltreated in childhood was also far more likely to experience subsequent traumatic events such as rape, physical assault, or other traumas. Additionally, the adult survivors of child abuse were significantly more likely to come from families with significant problems (parents being arrested, drugs or alcohol in self and family, early behavioral problems prior to abuse experiences, low level of education subsequent to abuse). These risk factors alone were found to be highly contributory to PTSD even in the absence of child abuse experiences. However, when correcting for the association of these variables, childhood sexual abuse was still associated with PTSD in adulthood but physical abuse and neglect were not. An analysis of the relationship between adult trauma and PTSD, controlling for childhood trauma, was not performed in this study.

Nishith et al. (2000) used path analysis to demonstrate that a history of child sexual abuse directly increased the vulnerability of adult and physical victimization and contributed substantially to current PTSD symptoms. This study is extremely important because it provides a solid basis for interpreting previous studies demonstrating current psychopathology among adults abused as children. The results of the path analysis, together with the extant literature on the effects of child abuse on revictimization and subsequent symptom development, clearly demonstrate a role for cumulative effects of childhood and subsequent traumatic events in the development of PTSD. Cumulative trauma appears to particularly account for the increased estimates of PTSD in adults with early childhood trauma relative to traumatized children. Given that the effects of early trauma are bound to initiate a progression of revictimization and symptoms, it is imperative to identify models that explain the cascade that culminates in complex psychopathology among those who experience untoward events when they are young, are revictimized, and show augmented and complex responses.

Biological Models of the Effects of Stress: The Centrality of Sensitization as a Mechanism of Permanent Stress Responses

Considerable interest was generated by early research on the physiologic effects of stress (Cannon 1914; Selye 1936, 1956). The initial studies as well as decades of confirmatory observations that followed led to the idea that external events could have a profound impact on the biology and behavior of organisms. Both acute and chronic stressors could have effects. However, critical to stress theory was that the stressor had to be present to exert its effects; once the stressor had been removed, the organism would begin a recovery from the effects of stress. In the 1970s and 1980s, a series of observations in laboratory animals led to the suggestion that the biological and behavioral effects of stress could continue and strengthen even after the stressor had been removed (Antelman 1988). In fact, exposure to even brief single-episode stressors, such as needle sticks, was demonstrated to have profound effects on how an animal would respond to a subsequent stressor (Antelman et al. 1991). The model of time-dependent sensitization and observations of kindled seizures that followed (reviewed in Post et al. 1997) laid the groundwork for current biobehavioral models of stress, which are grounded in the belief that some aspects of exposure can be permanent. These models provided a framework for understanding how traumatic events in humans could have biological and behavioral effects that persisted long after the termination of the event (Antelman et al. 1991; Post et al. 1997; Yehuda and Antelman 1993).

Indeed, molecular neurobiologic studies have demonstrated changes in the expression of genes that respond within minutes to environmental perturbations—observations that represent a remarkable paradigm shift from earlier formulations of the effects of stress. It is now clear that stress activates the formation of gene products, which in turn influence cellular processes that lead to gene expression, protein formation, and concomitant biological and behavioral change (Duman et al. 1994; Hyman and Nestler 1996). Thus, current stress theory is exceedingly focused on the lifelong implications of stressful experiences (McEwen and

Magarinos 1997), and investigators have become interested in examining biological cascades resulting from activation. Furthermore, the possibility of stress-induced changes in gene expression lays the groundwork for intergenerational effects of traumatic stress (Yehuda et al. 2000) and may eventually contribute to uncovering a genetic basis for individual differences in stress reactivity.

Against this backdrop, it becomes critically important to ask whether there may be differences in the long-term effects of stress depending on the developmental stage of an organism. Indeed, there is abundant evidence suggesting that adverse environmental events occurring early in life may differentially alter neurobiologic and behavioral systems and influence subsequent responses to stress, as reviewed below.

Developmental Influences of Early Stress in Animals

Early experiences are believed to set the level of responsiveness of the hypothalamic-pituitary-adrenal (HPA) axis and autonomic nervous system in such a way that these systems either overreact or underreact to stressful events (McEwen and Magarinos 1997). Indeed, different types of environmental experiences are associated with different neurobiologic outcomes. The elucidation of this biological heterogeneity may be critical to understanding individual differences in responses to early events.

Levine (1967) and Denenberg et al. (1967) were the first to show that exposure of infant animals to mild stress could permanently reduce the pituitary-adrenal responses to subsequent stressors in adulthood. These observations were replicated and further developed by Meaney et al. (1989), who showed that laboratory rats handled within the first 2 weeks of life showed significantly lower adrenocorticotropic hormone (ACTH) and corticosterone secretion at baseline and in response to stress in adulthood. Furthermore, early handled rats showed an enhanced cortisol suppression following dexamethasone, suggesting an enhanced negative feedback inhibition (Meaney et al. 1989). Consistent with these observations, studies of glucocorticoid receptor concentrations revealed an increased number of receptors (Meaney et al. 1988) and increased glucocorticoid receptor mRNA expression in the hippocampal tissue slices (Plotsky and Meaney 1993). The biological and behavioral findings noted above are similar to those observed in adolescents and adults with chronic PTSD—that is, low basal cortisol levels (Mason et al. 1986; Yehuda et al. 1990, 1993b, 1995c), increased cortisol response to dexamethasone (Kellner et al. 1997; M.B. Stein et al. 1997a; Yehuda et al. 1993a, 1995a), increased concentration of glucocorticoid receptor (Yehuda et al. 1993b, 1995a), and evidence of increased glucocorticoid receptor activity in the hippocampus (Grossman et al. 1999). However, there are some important differences between the biological consequences of early handling and those observed with PTSD in relation to corticotropin releasing factor (CRF) activity and subsequent neuroendocrine responses to stress. CRF appears to be elevated in PTSD (Baker et al. 1999) but not in early handled rats. Trauma survivors appear to show a pituitary-adrenocortical hyperresponsivity to stress (Heim et al. 2000), whereas early handled rats showed a lower response to stressors as well as a faster recovery to baseline.

Studies of laboratory rats exposed to maternal deprivation early in life appear to show a very different constellation of biological and behavioral changes than those receiving the manipulation of early handling (which only involves maternal separation for several minutes per day). In response to subsequent restraint or novelty stress, rats exposed to maternal deprivation show an increased cortisol and ACTH response (Plotsky and Meaney 1993). However, ACTH, but not cortisol concentrations, have been found to be elevated at baseline. Moreover, maternally deprived rats also showed a decreased cortisol response to dexamethasone and an increased expression of CRF mRNA expression in the hypothalamus (Ladd et al. 1996). Indeed, infant rats deprived of their mothers for a 24-hour period show increased CRF receptors in many other important brain regions, such as the frontal cortex, hippocampus, amygdala, and cerebellum, in addition to the hypothalamus. Therefore, the acute endocrine response to subsequent stress may result from biological sensitization due to prior alterations in CRF receptor regulation.

Studies of maternal deprivation in nonhuman primates have repeatedly pointed to the importance of early attachment in mediating individual differences in subsequent coping with adversity (Levine and Weiner 1988). Maternal deprivation in primates is certainly stressful, but it is not clear whether it is a better model for abuse or for neglect. Nonetheless, the response of monkeys deprived in infancy to subsequent stress cannot be predicted solely on the basis of this deprivation. Rather, temperamental, genetic, and environmental effects appear to be associated both with the monkey's ability to cope with environmental challenge as an adult and with variability in basal and stress-related changes in hormones such as ACTH and cortisol (Levine et al. 1993; Lyons et al. 2000).

Perhaps more relevant to studies of childhood stress are experiments of monkeys who were assigned to different rearing conditions in order to produce different types of foraging stress. In this paradigm, mothers and their infants were randomized into different rearing conditions requiring low (less stressful), higher (predictable stress), or variable (unpredictable, most stressful) foraging demands on the mother. The infant monkeys were subjected to these conditions until young adulthood (2–4 years), and then a series of biological tests were performed. Adult monkeys who had been reared in the variable foraging condition showed low cortisol but increased CRF levels (Coplan et al. 1996), similar to what has been observed in adults with chronic PTSD (Baker et al. 1999; Bremner et al. 1997a).

These studies in animals underscore the important role of early adverse life events in behavioral sensitization of both the HPA and noradrenergic systems. Although extrapolation from animal studies of stress to childhood traumatization is problematic, it is interesting to observe that neither the effects of childhood trauma nor early stressful life events in animals result in a uniform series of consequences but rather are predicted on the basis of a complex set of variables, including genetics, social interaction, and other mediating environmental events.

Biological Consequences in Adults Who Experienced Trauma in Childhood

Just as there are myriad behavioral and mental consequences associated with childhood traumatic experiences, there are likely to be a range of biological alterations associated with early trauma exposure. Indeed, the review above highlights that childhood maltreatment can be a risk factor for the development of many different mental conditions. To the extent that biological differences have been associated with these diverse outcomes, it could reasonably be assumed that there is no specific biological consequence related to early trauma. It is more reasonable to focus on the type of alterations that might be expected (e.g., neuroendocrine, neurochemical, neuroanatomic). To date, most studies examining long-term biological correlates of early abuse have done so in the context of either PTSD or major depression, and highlights from these studies are reviewed below. However, it would be important for future studies to examine the impact of early trauma as it occurs in adults in different diagnostic groups so that the breadth and scope of the biological sequelae of abuse can be related to the diversity of behavioral and symptomatic expression following such exposures.

Neurochemical and Neuroendocrine Findings in Adults Exposed to Childhood Maltreatment

Studies of PTSD in response to traumatic events occurring in adulthood (e.g., combat) have tended to show evidence for lower basal cortisol levels (Boscarino 1996; Yehuda et al. 1990, 1995c) and an enhanced negative feedback sensitivity of the HPA axis. This latter observation is supported by findings of increased cortisol suppression following low doses of dexamethasone (Yehuda et al. 1993a, 1995a). This finding is in the opposite direction of the nonsuppression following dexamethasone observed in studies of depression. Interestingly, in many (but not all) studies, adults with PTSD were also found to show evidence of increased catecholamine activity (e.g., Yehuda et al. 1998; also reviewed in Southwick et al. 1993).

Indeed, this profile was similarly observed in adolescents with PTSD who were exposed to a devastating earthquake in Armenia. Subjects with PTSD showed elevated levels of salivary MHPG (3-methoxy-4-hydroxyphenylglycol) and reduced concentrations of salivary cortisol. Subjects with PTSD also showed an enhanced suppression of cortisol after low-dose dexamethasone (0.50 mg) (Goenjian et al. 1996). Both basal MHPG levels and the response to dexamethasone were correlated with symptoms in the PTSD group.

The results of studies examining survivors of childhood maltreatment have been more contradictory. Lemieux and Coe (1995) showed that, in a sample of women who were survivors of childhood sexual abuse, those with PTSD had significantly elevated cortisol, norepinephrine, and epinephrine levels compared with those without PTSD. Common to both groups of abused women was the finding of increased polyuria, increased vaginal discomfort and infection, and increased menstrual difficulty. Abused subjects in that study also tended to be more obese, particularly if they had PTSD, which might, in part, contribute to higher ambient hormone levels. Studies of maltreated children with PTSD have also demonstrated slight elevations in cortisol and catecholamines compared with normal control subjects (De Bellis et al. 2000). In contrast, Stein et al. (1997b) reported that women who survived childhood sexual abuse displayed an enhanced suppression of cortisol following dexamethasone, similar to what has been observed in other groups of survivors with PTSD. These authors also found an (insignificant) increase in lymphocyte glucocorticoid receptor number. Thus, although there are similarities in the HPA axis abnormalities associated with PTSD due to childhood abuse and adult traumatization, further work is needed to understand the differences and their relationship to type of trauma, development, and longitudinal course.

Stress Reactivity in Adults Exposed to Childhood Maltreatment

Studies of adults abused as children suggest a greater stress reactivity, both behaviorally and biologically. For example, in a sample of 491 female college students screened for sexual abuse, women with a history of childhood sexual abuse were found to display stronger emotional responses to everyday daily hassles and stressors compared with those sexually abused in adulthood or not abused (Thakkar and McCanne 2000). Correspondingly, Heim et al. (2000) reported exaggerated pituitary-adrenal and autonomic responses to stress in women with childhood physical and sexual abuse. The responses of 13 women with depression and childhood sexual abuse, 14 women with childhood physical and sexual abuse without depression, 10 women with depression but without childhood abuse, and 12 comparison subjects were compared on measures of biological reactivity in response to a psychologic stressor. Women with early abuse demonstrated an exaggerated ACTH response to the stressor, particularly if they also met the diagnostic criteria for major depression. These findings suggest that the HPA axis is more responsive to stress in symptomatic survivors of trauma, as implied by studies demonstrating an enhanced circadian rhythmicity (Yehuda et al. 1996) and exaggerated negative feedback inhibition (Yehuda et al. 1995a) in PTSD.

Neuroanatomic Studies in Adults Exposed to Childhood Maltreatment

It has been of interest to specifically examine the brain regions involved in emotion and stress responses (e.g., the medial prefrontal cortex, amygdala, and hippocampus) in trauma survivors to obtain an understanding of the emotional and biological consequences of traumatic stress exposure. The medial prefrontal dopaminergic system is particularly sensitive to stress and appears to influence cortisol and sympathetic responses to stress. Activation of this area also inhibits the fear responses of the amygdala in animals exposed to threat. The amygdala plays a pivotal role in the expression of fear and anxiety and works in tandem with the hippocampus to assess immediate threat and process the memory of such threats. Also involved in information processing of threat-related stimuli are structures related to the anterolateral prefrontal cortex, including the posterior cingulate, parietal and motor cortex, and cerebellum. Accordingly, alterations in brain metabolism have been found in these areas in adult trauma survivors with PTSD (Bremner et al. 1997b; Rauch et al. 1996, 2000; Semple et al. 1996). Because numerous brain regions are involved in emotional processing and stress, some functional imaging studies have used statistical probability mapping rather than specifying particular regions of interest. As such, these techniques examine the relationship between brain function and behavior, examining the entire brain. Significant changes in metabolism are noted that may explain the pathophysiology of the disorder.

Of particular interest are those studies that have shown that the anterior cingulate is less active in trauma-exposed subjects with PTSD. Reduced blood flow to the anterior cingulate following script-driven imagery has been described in adult women with PTSD as a result of sexual abuse in childhood ($n=10$) compared with similarly traumatized women who did not meet criteria for PTSD ($n=12$) (Bremner et al. 1999; Shin et al. 1999). Similarly, a lower level of blood flow to the anterior cingulate has been described in Vietnam War veterans with PTSD in response to combat-related stimuli (Bremner et al. 1999). Using proton magnetic resonance spectroscopy, a reduced ratio of N-acetylaspartate and creatinine was found in the anterior cingulate of 11 children and adolescents with PTSD following child abuse compared with 11 healthy control subjects (De Bellis et al. 2000). The anterior cingulate is thought to exert an inhibitory effect on the amygdala and other regions involved in the fear response. Together, these studies suggest that aspects of PTSD may result from a disinhibition of the amygdala due to reduced anterior cingulate activity, which may then promote fear conditioning and continuation of a fear response even in the absence of a fear stimulus.

Examination of hippocampal volume using magnetic resonance imaging has also provided evidence for a smaller hippocampal volume in adult survivors of childhood trauma. The hippocampus has been of particular interest in PTSD because of its critical role in learning and memory and its sensitivity to stress hormones. An initial report demonstrated smaller hippocampal volumes in 17 men and women adult survivors of child abuse compared with 17 nonabused control subjects (Bremner et al. 1995). However, insofar as all exposed subjects had current and lifetime PTSD, it was not possible to determine whether this was an effect of trauma or PTSD. Indeed, because Gurvits et al. (1996) demonstrated a smaller hippocampal volume in seven Vietnam War veterans with PTSD compared with seven veterans without PTSD, it may be reasonable to conclude that the effects observed are associated with PTSD. On the other hand, these authors reported a negative correlation between hippocampal volume and trauma exposure, which suggests severity of exposure is relevant to this finding. M.B. Stein et al. (1997b) showed reduced hippocampal volume in a sample of 21 women who had been severely sexually abused in childhood, of whom 15 met the diagnostic criteria for PTSD. The other subjects met criteria for dissociative or other disorders associated with childhood sexual abuse. Although the results of these studies are intriguing, most subjects with PTSD in the aforementioned studies also had multiple comorbid psychiatric disorders, including, most notably, alcohol and substance abuse. Because substance abuse is associated with hippocampal volume loss in and of itself (De Bellis et al. 2000; Laasko et al. 2000), it remains unclear to what extent the results reflect comorbid substance abuse. Further work is needed to understand whether the smaller hippocampal volumes in PTSD represent a risk factor for or consequence of trauma exposure, PTSD, or associated comorbidities.

De Bellis et al. (1999) have recently demonstrated a diffuse loss of brain size but not smaller hippocampal volumes in children who have been maltreated. They argued that the effects of early abuse may affect multiple systems, and thus the entire brain, because postnatal development occurs ubiquitously in brain. Teicher et al. (1996) argued that although all aspects of brain development may be affected by early abuse, some areas may be particularly vulnerable. In addition to the hippocampus, amygdala, prefrontal cortex, and other limbic areas, they hypothesized that early abuse adversely affects the development of the corpus callosum and hemispheric integration and dominance.

To examine potential relationships between early abuse and limbic system dysfunction, Teicher et al. (1993) devised a questionnaire that measured symptoms often encountered in temporal lobe epilepsy. These items consisted primarily of paroxysmal somatic disturbances, brief hallucinatory events, visual phenomena, automatisms, and dissociative experiences. Among subjects who presented for outpatient psychiatric treatment, adults who endorsed both physical and sexual abuse ($n=41$) scored more than twice as high as subjects who were never abused ($n=109$) (Teicher et al. 1996). In a chart review of 115 consecutive admissions to a child and adolescent psychiatric hospital, evidence of neurologic abnormalities was investigated. Subjects with frank neurologic disturbance were omitted from analyses. In the remaining subjects ($n=104$), the authors found that 60% of subjects with physical and or sexual abuse had abnormal electroencephalographic findings compared with 43% of subjects with no abuse. Left-hemisphere deficits were more than twice as likely to be present in abused subjects (Teicher et al. 1996).

The model developed by Teicher et al. (1996) is one in which early abuse leads to myriad developmental brain abnormalities. These abnormalities further potentiate the negative effects of neurohormonal release in response to negative environmental events. For example, to the extent that neuronal inputs to various brain regions are affected by abuse, this can give rise to anxiogenic, amnestic, somatic, or dissociative effects and initiate a cascade that involves further neurochemical and behavioral disruption. The precise nature of the consequences of abuse is a function of the developmental processes that are disrupted as well as further events that occur. As different brain regions lose function and show an increased tendency toward reduced rather than increased hemispheric interconnectivity, cognitive capacities are further affected that may lay the groundwork for deficits in cognitive processing in adults associated with trauma-related disorders.

PTSD and Other Psychological Symptoms in Adults Who Survived the Holocaust as Children

The previous sections highlight the long-term impact of maltreatment in childhood on behavior and biology and underscore differences between experiences such as sexual abuse, physical abuse, and chronic neglect as well as single-episode events such as disasters and violent events that are clearly unusual in the scope of a child's life. The primary differences in the effects of these types of trauma appear to be related to the degree of recovery and the breadth of symptomatology. Data are lacking regarding the frequency of revictimization and long-term biological impairment in adults who survived single-episode traumatic events.

Although the DSM-IV acknowledges that chronic PTSD can develop after either single-episode or chronic traumatic events, it is clear that the overall consequences of single versus chronic events may be quite different, as described by Terr (1991). Creating a dichotomy between single and chronic exposure based on comparing single-episode traumas with child abuse, however, does not fully capture the range of potentially life-altering experiences that can occur. Indeed, there are multiple different types of chronic traumatic stressors that are not the result of either social disadvantage or repeated physical or sexual abuse, for example, children who are exposed to war, ethnic cleansing, political oppression, concomitant interpersonal violence, and flight from their homes. It is not currently known whether the long-lasting impact of these events can be more likened to single-episode traumas (which are associated with a greater degree of recovery) or child maltreatment involving physical and sexual abuse (which are associated with the more complex, diverse, and enduring outcomes).

In the context of this question, it is compelling to examine the long-term consequences of child survivors of war. In recent years, investigators have begun to describe the mental health ramifications of having experienced the Holocaust in childhood. The Holocaust was inarguably an isolated experience in the lives of its survivors but one that lasted over a period of several years for most. The "risk factor" for exposure to this event was being Jewish in Europe. In response to the threat of annihilation, many attempted to flee. Those who were not interned in camps nonetheless experienced traumas including being beaten or tortured, witnessing torture and murder, having to survive in hiding, assuming a false identity, and fleeing under threat of death. Some children experienced one or more of these events without their parents. The evaluation of Holocaust survivors affords an opportunity to examine the long-term effects of an event that is of comparable magnitude to physical and sexual abuse. Because the Holocaust occurred during a discrete period in history and its victims were of different ages, it is further possible to evaluate differential responses to this event based on the stage of development.

In our sample of community-dwelling Holocaust survivors, which included survivors who were in camps as well as those who were in hiding, we have found that nearly half continue to suffer from PTSD despite the passage of more than 50 years. Indeed, despite the differences in the types of traumas experienced by those in camps as opposed to those in hiding, these groups did not differ considerably in types of symptoms. There were, however, considerable differences based on the age of trauma exposure. Particularly marked in the younger survivors were hypervigilance, psychogenic amnesia, emotional detachment, and dissociation (Yehuda et al. 1997). Subjects who were younger during the Holocaust were also likely to show greater psychopathology on a range of symptoms on the Symptom Checklist-90 (Derogatis 1983). Similar to what has been described in victims of child maltreatment, current PTSD symptoms in Holocaust survivors were significantly associated with cumulative lifetime trauma (Yehuda et al. 1995b). Thus, in this group of survivors who were exposed early in life to extreme trauma but not at the hands of family or other caretakers, the mental health consequences of such trauma appear to be severe, persistent, and related to developmental stage at the time of traumatization.

Methodologic Considerations in the Study of the Long-Term Impact of Childhood Trauma

Most of what we know about the impact of childhood trauma has come from retrospective reports. These studies are vulnerable because of their reliance on subjective data from people who may or may not have accurate recall of remote events and whose memories cannot be corroborated independently. Indeed, it has been repeatedly demonstrated that human memory for traumatic events is not reliable. In some cases, people appear to have recall for events that never happened and in other cases forget traumatic things that clearly did happen. In either situation, it is usually difficult for a third party to know whether any claim or denial of abuse is the truth. Additionally, because most studies have been performed on convenience samples (mostly those suspected of having experienced abuse or who have a disproportionately high level of mental health or behavioral problems), a question arises about the generalizability of such studies.

Some reports have demonstrated a lack of correlation between disclosure of abuse and consequences when evaluated prospectively versus retrospectively (J. Brown et al. 1998; Widom et al. 1999). Thus, it may be that retrospective studies overestimate the range and severity of consequences relating to past abuse. This problem is further compounded if studies rely heavily on data from clinical populations. However, the issue of generalization and bias relating to retrospective clinical observation may be less relevant in a clinical situation than in other arenas, such as policy and law, in which this information is often used.

Certainly, the formulation of assumptions about the long-term impact of abuse on the basis of such retrospective clinical studies may constitute a problem for policymakers, social advocates, or attorneys trying to prove or disprove facts in a court of law. However, when applied to issues in clinical treatment, the retrospective and subjective accounts of early events are quite relevant. In clinical practice, it is the retrospective report of trauma that appears to be most associated with a high likelihood of morbidity in patients. Thus, to the extent that there are discrepancies between prospective and retrospective evaluations, these approaches may bear on questions that are particularly relevant in different settings. The association between retrospective recollections and certain consequences is highly relevant for the practicing clinician who relies on this kind of information for the purpose of better understanding a patient. On the other hand, prospective studies are essential for the needs of the policymaker who is in charge of allocation of resources for the treatment of the consequences of abuse.

Other methodologic issues in the literature, such as a failure to control for demographic and other background variables that might increase the likelihood of both victimization and psychologic symptoms, may also obfuscate a clear understanding of the relationship between early events and subsequent pathology. Co-occurrences of various types of victimization and assumptions that a given symptom is a result of victimization rather than a risk factor are potentially greater problems for the field than is retrospective bias. Indeed, approaches taken by investigators such as Briere et al. (1997) are critical if the field is indeed to elucidate connections between psychological sequelae and childhood sexual abuse after controlling for other factors associated with abuse. Indeed, a failure to control for relevant variables may completely obscure any associations between trauma and its consequences.

Retrospective evaluation of the association between trauma exposure and its supposed consequences may be biased in that people's recollections of traumatic events may well be influenced by the consequences of adversity. A patient who has nightmares because of abuse may be more likely to report that abuse occurred than a patient who does not experience symptoms. Thus, the apparent association between abuse and nightmares may not hold true in a prospective evaluation. However, in clinical practice, this association would be highly significant. This point can be illustrated in a study by Hunter and Kilstrom (1979) that asked mothers of newly born children about their own history of abuse and then reevaluated the mothers after 1 year. A strong link between retrospectively reported maternal history of abuse and child maltreatment was found (9 of 10 maltreating mothers reported having been abused themselves at the 1-year follow-up) but this association was much weaker in the prospective analysis of the same cohort (9 of 49). This finding suggests that recollections of traumatic events are biased but are often based on responses to environmental circumstances that provide salience. Disclosure of memories of abuse may be more likely to be triggered in the context of particular current events and may be best discussed in that context. Because adult survivors of early abuse are more likely to be retraumatized, the negative consequences of the past seem to be literally sustained and amplified by subsequent traumas, thus creating a vicious circle in which the return to homeostasis and recovery becomes increasingly challenging from a psychologic and biological perspective.

Summary and Conclusions

The effects of childhood maltreatment on adults are diverse and include, but are not limited to, mental disorders such as PTSD, depression, anxiety disorders, interpersonal difficulties, and medical problems. Most of what is known about the psychologic and biological effects of early maltreatment comes from retrospective studies of clinical samples. The use of retrospective studies in clinical samples raises issues about the generalizability of the findings, the veracity of recall, and the influence of current experiences and symptoms on the selectivity of recall. Nonetheless, it appears clear from this substantial literature that perhaps one of the most harmful outcomes of child maltreatment is that it substantially increases the risk of subsequent victimization. This retraumatization and the additive biological and behavioral outcomes of subsequent events appear to sustain, perpetuate, and amplify symptomatology of those exposed to trauma in childhood.

Several major gaps exist in our knowledge at this time. There is a need to better delineate the additional risk factors that mediate disease and recovery from abuse, the relationship between the biological and behavioral consequences of abuse, and the similarities and differences between the consequences of exposure to single and multiple traumas and between interpersonal trauma and other types of trauma and their cumulative effects. It is necessary to identify which environmental factors exacerbate and which reduce the effects of stress and likelihood of revictimization and to examine the impact of altering environments appropriately for children who have been exposed to trauma. It is hoped that as the consequences of abuse become clearer, it will be possible to provide more focused interventions for both the abused child and the adult suffering from the effects of such exposures.

References

Alexander PC, Lupfer SL: Family characteristics and long-term consequences associated with sexual abuse. Arch Sex Behav 16:235–245, 1987

American Psychiatric Association: Diagnostic and Statistical Manual of Mental Disorders, 4th Edition. Washington, DC, American Psychiatric Association, 1994

Antelman SM: Time-dependent sensitization as the cornerstone for a new approach to pharmacotherapy: drugs as foreign/stressful stimuli. Drug Dev Res 14:1–30, 1988

Antelman SM, Caggiula AR, Kocan D, et al: One experience with "lower" or "higher" intensity stressors, respectively enhances or diminishes responsiveness to haloperidol weeks later: implications for understanding drug variability. Brain Res 566:276–283, 1991

Bagley C, Ramsay R: Sexual abuse in childhood: psychosocial outcomes and implications for social work practice. Journal of Social Work and Human Sexuality 4:33–47, 1986

Baker DG, West SA, Nicholson WE, et al: Serial CSF corticotropin-releasing hormone levels and adrenocortical activity in combat veterans with posttraumatic stress disorder. Am J Psychiatry 156:585–588, 1999

Beitchman JH, Zucker KJ, Hood JE, et al: A review of the long-term effects of child abuse. Child Abuse Negl 16:101–118, 1992

Boscarino JA: Posttraumatic stress disorder, exposure to combat, and lower plasma cortisol among Vietnam veterans: findings and clinical implications. J Consult Clin Psychol 64:191–201, 1996

Boudewyn AC, Liem JH: Childhood sexual abuse as a precursor to depression and self-destructive behavior in adulthood. J Trauma Stress 8:445–459, 1995

Bremner JD, Southwick SM, Johnsons DR, et al: Childhood physical abuse and combat-related posttraumatic stress disorder in Vietnam veterans. Am J Psychiatry 150:235–239, 1993

Bremner JD, Randall P, Scott TM, et al: MRI-based measurement of hippocampal volume in patients with combat-related posttraumatic stress disorder. Am J Psychiatry 152:973–981, 1995

Bremner JD, Licinoio J, Darnell A, et al: Elevated CSF corticotropin-releasing factor concentrations in posttraumatic stress disorder. Am J Psychiatry 154:624–629, 1997a

Bremner JD, Randall P, Vermetten E, et al: Magnetic resonance imaging-based measurement of hippocampal volume in posttraumatic stress disorder related to childhood physical and sexual abuse: a preliminary report. Biol Psychiatry 41:23–32, 1997b

Bremner JD, Narayan M, Staib LH, et al: Neural correlates of memories of childhood sexual abuse in women with and without posttraumatic stress disorder. Am J Psychiatry 156:1787–1795, 1999

Briere J: The long-term clinical correlates of childhood sexual victimization. Ann N Y Acad Sci 528:327–334, 1988

Briere JN, Elliot DM: Immediate and long-term impacts of child sexual abuse. Future Child 4:54–69, 1994

Briere J, Runtz M: Post-sexual abuse trauma: data and implications for clinical practice. Journal of Interpersonal Violence 2:367–379, 1987

Briere J, Runtz M: Multivariate correlates of childhood psychological and physical maltreatment among university women. Child Abuse Negl 12:331–341, 1988

Briere J, Runtz M: The long-term effects of sexual abuse: a review and synthesis. New Directions in Mental Health Services 51:3–13, 1991

Briere J, Evans D, Runtz M, et al: Symptomatology in men who were molested as children: a comparison study. Am J Orthopsychiatry 53: 457–461, 1988

Briere J, Woo R, McRae B, et al: Lifetime victimization history, demographics, and clinical status in female psychiatric emergency room patients. J Nerv Ment Dis 185:95–101, 1997

Briggs L, Joyce PR: What determines post-traumatic stress disorder symptomatology for survivors of childhood sexual abuse? Child Abuse Negl 21:575–582, 1997

Brown GR, Anderson B: Psychiatric morbidity in adult inpatients with childhood histories of sexual and physical abuse. Am J Psychiatry 148:55–61, 1991

Brown J, Cohen P, Johnson JG, et al: A longitudinal analysis of risk factors for child maltreatment findings of a 17-year prospective study of officially recorded and self-reported child abuse and neglect. Child Abuse Negl 22:1065–1078, 1998

Browne A, Finkelhor D: Impact of child sexual abuse: a review of the research. Psychol Bull 99:66–77, 1986

Brunngraber LS: Father-daughter incest: immediate and long-term effects of sexual abuse. Adv Nurs Sci 8:15–35, 1986

Bryer JB, Nelson BA, Miller JB, et al: Childhood sexual and physical abuse as factors in adult psychiatric illness. Am J Psychiatry 144: 1426–1430, 1987

Bushnell JA, Wells JE, Oakley-Browne MA: Long-term effects of intrafamilial sexual abuse in childhood. Acta Psychiatr Scand 85:136–142, 1992

Cahill C, Llewelyn SP, Pearson C: Long-term effects of sexual abuse which occurred in childhood: a review. Br J Clin Psychol 30:117–130, 1991

Cannon WB: Emergency function of adrenal medulla in pain and major emotions. Am J Physiol 3:356–372, 1914

Chu JA, Dill DL: Dissociative symptoms in relation to childhood physical and sexual abuse. Am J Psychiatry 147:887–893, 1990

Cloitre M, Tardiff K, Marzuk PM, et al: Childhood abuse and subsequent sexual assault among female inpatients. J Trauma Stress 9:473–482, 1996

Cloitre M, Scarvalone P, Difede J: Posttraumatic stress disorder, self- and interpersonal dysfunction among sexually retraumatized women. J Trauma Stress 10:437–452, 1997

Collings SJ: The long-term effects of contact and noncontact forms of child sexual abuse in a sample of university men. Child Abuse Negl 19:1–6, 1995

Coplan JD, Andrews MW, Rosenblum LA, et al: Persistent elevations of cerebrospinal fluid concentrations of corticotropin-releasing factor in adult nonhuman primates exposed to early life stressors: implications for the pathophysiology of mood and anxiety disorders. Proc Natl Acad Sci U S A 93:1619–1623, 1996

Dancu CV, Riggs DS, Hearst-Ikeda D, et al: Dissociative experiences and posttraumatic stress disorder among female victims of criminal assault and rape. J Trauma Stress 9:253–267, 1996

De Bellis MD, Baum AS, Birmaher B, et al: A.E. Bennett Research Award. Developmental traumatology, part I: biological stress systems. Biol Psychiatry 45:1259–1270, 1999

De Bellis MD, Clark DB, Beers SR, et al: Hippocampal volume in adolescent-onset alcohol use disorders. Am J Psychiatry 157:737–744, 2000

Deblinger E, McLeer SV, Atkins MS, et al: Posttraumatic stress in sexually abused, physically abused and non-abused children. Child Abuse Negl 13:403–408, 1989

Denenberg VH, Brumaghim JT, Haltmeyer GC, et al: Increased adrenocortical activity in the neonatal rat following handling. Endocrinology 81:1047–1052, 1967

DePaul J, Domenech L: Childhood history of abuse and child abuse potential in adolescent mothers: a longitudinal study. Child Abuse Negl 24:701–713, 2000

Derogatis LR: SCL-90-R administration: scoring and procedures manual II. Towson, MD, Clinical Psychometric Research, 1983

Desivilya HS, Gal R, Ayalon O: Extent of victimization, traumatic stress symptoms, and adjustment of terrorist assault survivors: a long-term follow-up. J Trauma Stress 9:881–889, 1996

Duman RS, Heninger GR, Nestler EJ: Molecular psychiatry: adaptations of receptor-coupled signal transduction pathways underlying stress- and drug-induced neural plasticity. J Nerv Ment Dis 182:692–700, 1994

Ellason JW, Ross CA, Sainton K, et al: Axis I and II comorbidity and childhood trauma history in chemical dependency. Bull Menninger Clin 60:39–51, 1996

Elliot DM, Briere J: Posttraumatic stress associated with delayed recall of sexual abuse: a general population study. J Trauma Stress 8:629–647, 1995

Ellis E, Atkeson BM, Calhoun K: An examination of differences between multiple and single-incident victims of sexual assault. J Abnorm Psychol 91:221–224, 1982

Epstein JN, Saunders BE, Kilpatrick DG: Predicting PTSD in women with a history of childhood rape. J Trauma Stress 10:573–587, 1997

Epstein JN, Saunders BE, Kilpatrick DG, et al: PTSD as a mediator between childhood rape and alcohol use in adult women. Child Abuse Negl 22:223–234, 1998

Felitti VJ: Long-term medical consequences of incest, rape, and molestation. South Med J 84:328–331, 1991

Finkelhor D: Sexually Victimized Children. New York, Free Press, 1979

Fleming J, Mujllen PE, Sibthorpe B, et al: The long-term impact of childhood sexual abuse in Australian women. Child Abuse Negl 23:145–159, 1999

Follette VM, Polusny MA, Milbeck K: Mental health and law enforcement professionals: trauma history, psychological symptoms, and impact of providing service to child sexual abuse survivors. Professional Psychology: Research and Practice 25:275–282, 1994

Follette VM, Polusny MA, Bechtle AE, et al: Cumulative trauma: the impact of child sexual abuse, adult sexual assault and spouse abuse. J Trauma Stress 9:25–35, 1996

Fromuth ME: The relationship of childhood sexual abuse with later psychological and sexual adjustment in a sample of college women. Child Abuse Negl 10:5–15, 1986

Fromuth ME, Burkhart BR: Long-term psychological correlates of childhood sexual abuse in two samples of college men. Child Abuse Negl 13:533–542, 1989

Garrison C, Bryant E, Addy C, et al: Posttraumatic stress disorder in adolescents after Hurricane Andrew. J Am Acad Child Adolesc Psychiatry 34:1193–1201, 1995

Gelinas DJ: The persisting negative effects of incest. Psychiatry 46:312–332, 1983

Gidycz CA, Coble CN, Latham L, et al: Sexual assault experience in adulthood and prior victimization experiences: a prospective analysis. Psychology of Women Quarterly 17:151–168, 1993

Gleser GC, Green BL, Winget C: Prolonged Psychosocial Effects of Disaster: A Study of Buffalo Creek. New York, Academic Press, 1981

Goenjian AK, Yehuda R, Pynoos RS, et al: Basal cortisol, dexamethasone suppression of cortisol, and MHP adolescents after the 1988 earthquake in Armenia. Am J Psychiatry 153:929–934, 1996

Gold ER: Long-term effects of sexual victimization in childhood: an attributional approach. J Consult Clin Psychol 54:471–475, 1986

Gorcey M, Santiago JM, McCall-Perez F: Psychological consequences for women sexually abused in childhood. Social Psychiatry 21:129–133, 1986

Green AH: Child sexual abuse: immediate and long-term effects and intervention. J Am Acad Child Adolesc Psychiatry 32:890–902, 1993

Green BL, Korol M, Grace MC, et al: Children and disaster: age, gender, and parental effects on PTSD symptoms. J Am Acad Child Adolesc Psychiatry 30:945–951, 1991

Green BL, Grace MC, Vary MG, et al: Children of disaster in the second decade: a 17-year follow-up of Buffalo Creek Survivors. J Am Acad Child Adolesc Psychiatry 33:71–79, 1994

Greenwald E, Leitenberg H, Cado S, et al: Childhood sexual abuse: long-term effects on psychological and sexual functioning in a nonclinical and nonstudent sample of adult women. Child Abuse Negl 14:503–513, 1990

Grossman R, Yehuda R, Buchsbaum M: [18]FDG PET neuroimaging following hydrocortisone infusion in PTSD. Presented at the 1999 ISTSS Meeting, Miami, FL, November, 1999

Gurvits TG, Shenton MR, Hokama H, et al: Magnetic resonance imaging study of hippocampal volume in chronic combat-related posttraumatic stress disorder. Biol Psychiatry 40: 192–199, 1996

Harter S, Alexander PC: Long-term effects of incestuous child abuse in college women: social adjustment, social cognition, and family characteristics. J Consult Clin Psychol 56:5–8, 1988

Heim C, Newport DJ, Heit S, et al: Pituitary-adrenal and autonomic responses to stress in women after sexual and physical abuse. JAMA 284:592–597, 2000

Herman JL: Father–Daughter Incest. Cambridge, MA, Harvard University Press, 1981

Herman JL, Schatzow E: Recovery and verification of memories of childhood sexual trauma. Psychoanalytic Psychology 4:1–14, 1987

Horowitz K, Weine S, Jekel J: PTSD symptoms in urban adolescent girls: compounded community trauma. J Am Acad Child Adolesc Psychiatry 34:1353–1361, 1995

Hunter RS, Kilstrom N: Breaking the cycle in abusive families. Am J Psychiatry 136:1320–1322, 1979

Hyman SE, Nestler EJ: Initiation and adaptation: a paradigm for understanding psychotropic drug action. Am J Psychiatry 153:151–162, 1996

Johnson JG, Smailes EM, Phil M, et al: Associations between four types of childhood neglect and personality disorder symptoms during adolescence and early adulthood: findings of a community-based longitudinal study. Journal of Personality Disorders 14:171–187, 2000

Kellner M, Baker DG, Yehuda R: Salivary cortisol in Operation Desert Storm returnees. Biol Psychiatry 42:849–850, 1997

Kendall-Tackett KA, Simon AF: Molestation and the onset of puberty: data from 365 adults molested as children. Child Abuse Negl 12:73–81, 1988

Kendall-Tackett KA, Williams LM, Finkelhor D: Impact of sexual abuse on children: a review and synthesis of recent empirical studies. Psychol Bull 113:164–180, 1993

Kinzie J, Sack W, Angell R, et al: The psychiatric effects of massive trauma on Cambodian children. J Am Acad Child Adolesc Psychiatry 25:370–376, 1986

Kiser LJ, Heston J, Millsap PA, et al: Physical and sexual abuse in childhood: relationship with posttraumatic stress disorder. J Am Acad Child Adolesc Psychiatry 30:776–783, 1991

Koss MP, Dinero TE: Discriminant analysis of risk factors for sexual victimization among a national sample of college women. J Consult Clin Psychol 57:242–250, 1989

Kunitz SJ, Levy JE, McCloskey J, et al: Alcohol dependence and domestic violence as sequelae of abuse and conduct disorder in childhood. Child Abuse Negl 22:1079–1091, 1998

Laasko MP, Vaurio O, Savolainen L, et al: A volumetric MRI study of the hippocampus in type 1 and 2 alcoholism. Behav Brain Res 109:177–186, 2000

Ladd CO, Owens MJ, Nemeroff CB: Persistent changes in corticotropin-releasing factor neuronal systems induced by maternal deprivation. Endocrinology 137:1212–1218, 1996

Laor N, Wolmer L, Mayes LC, et al: Israeli preschool children under Scuds: a 30 month follow-up. J Am Acad Child Adolesc Psychiatry 36:349–356, 1997

Lawrence KJ, Cozolino L, Foy DW: Psychological sequelae in adult females reporting childhood ritualistic abuse. Child Abuse Negl 19:975–984, 1995

Lemieux AM, Coe CL: Abuse-related posttraumatic stress disorder: evidence for chronic neuroendocrine activation in women. Psychosom Med 57:105–115, 1995

Levine S: Maternal and environmental influences on the adrenocortical response to stress in weanling rats. Science 14:258–260, 1967

Levine S, Weiner SG: Psychoendocrine aspects of mother-infant relationships in nonhuman primates. Psychoneuroendocrinology 13: 143–154, 1988

Levine S, Weiner SG, Coe CL: Temporal and social factors influencing behavioral and hormonal responses to separation in mother and infant squirrel monkeys. Psychoneuroendocrinology 18:297–306, 1993

Lindberg FH, Distad LJ: Post-traumatic stress disorders in women who experienced childhood incest. Child Abuse Negl 9:329–334, 1985

Luntz BK, Widom CS: Antisocial personality disorder in abused and neglected children grown up. Am J Psychiatry 151:670–674, 1994

Lyons DM, Yang C, Mobley BW, et al: Early environmental regulation of glucocorticoid feedback sensitivity in young adult monkeys. J Neuroendocrinol 12:723–728, 2000

Malinsky-Rummell R, Hansen DJ: Long-term consequences of childhood physical abuse. Psychol Bull 114:68–79, 1993

Mancini C, Van Ameringen M, MacMillan H: Relationship of childhood sexual and physical abuse to anxiety disorders. J Nerv Ment Dis 183:309–314, 1995

Marhoefer-Dvorak S, Resick PA, Hutter CK, et al: Single-versus multiple-incident rape victims: a comparison of psychological reactions to rape. Journal of Interpersonal Violence 3:145–160, 1988

Mason JW, Giller EL, Kosten TR, et al: Urinary free-cortisol levels in posttraumatic stress disorder patients. J Nerv Ment Dis 174:145–149, 1986

McCauley J, Kern D, Kolodner K, et al: Clinical characteristics of women with a history of childhood abuse: unhealed wounds. JAMA 277:1362–1368, 1997

McEwen BS, Magarinos AM: Stress effects on morphology and function of the hippocampus. Ann N Y Acad Sci 821:271–284, 1997

McNew JA, Abell N: Posttraumatic stress symptomatology: similarities and difference between Vietnam veterans and adult survivors of childhood sex abuse. Soc Work 40:115–126, 1995

Meaney M, Aitken D, Berkel H, et al: Effect of neonatal handling of age-related impairments associated with the hippocampus. Science 239:766–768, 1988

Meaney MJ, Aitken DH, Viau V, et al: Neonatal handling alters adreno-cortical negative feedback sensitivity and hippocampal type II gluco-corticoid receptor binding in the rat. Neuroendocrinology 50:597–604, 1989

Meiselman KC: Incest: A Psychological Study of Causes and Effects with Treatment Recommendations. San Francisco, CA, Josey Bass, 1978

Merrill LL, Newell CE, Thomsen CJ, et al: Childhood abuse and sexual revictimization in a female navy recruit sample. J Trauma Stress 12: 211–225, 1999

Moeller TP, Bachmann GA, Moeller JR: The combined effects of physical, sexual and emotional abuse during childhood: long-term consequences for women. Child Abuse Negl 17:623–640, 1993

Mullen PE, Martin JL, Anderson JC, et al: The long-term impact of the physical, emotional, and sexual abuse of children: a community study. Child Abuse Negl 20:7–21, 1996

Nash MR, Hulsey TL, Sexton MC, et al: Long-term sequelae of childhood sexual abuse: perceived family environment, psychopathology, and dissociation. J Consult Clin Psychol 61:276–283, 1993

Nishith P, Mechanic MB, Resick PA: Prior interpersonal trauma: the contribution to current PTSD symptoms in female rape victims. J Abnorm Psychol 109:20–25, 2000

Norris FH, Kaniasty K: Psychological distress following criminal victimization in the general population: cross-sectional, longitudinal, and prospective analyses. J Consult Clin Psychol 62:111–123, 1994

Peters SD: Child sexual abuse and later psychological problems, in Lasting Effects of Child Sexual Abuse. Edited by Wyatt GE, Powell GJ. Newbury Park, CA, Sage Publications, 1988, pp 101–117

Plotsky PM, Meaney MJ: Early, postnatal experience alters hypothalamic corticotropin-releasing factor (CRF) mRNA, median eminence CRF content a stress-induced release in adult rats. Brain Res Mol Brain Res 18:195–200, 1993

Post RM, Weiss SRB, Smith M, et al: Kindling versus quenching: implications for the evolution and treatment of posttraumatic stress disorder. Ann N Y Acad Sci 821:285–295, 1997

Pynoos R, Frederick C, Nader K, et al: Life threat and posttraumatic stress in school-age children. Arch Gen Psychiatry 44:1057–1063, 1987

Raczek SW: Childhood abuse and personality disorders. Journal of Personality Disorders 6:109–116, 1992

Rauch SL, van der Kolk, BA, Fisler RE, et al: A symptom provocation study of posttraumatic stress disorder using positron emission tomography and script-driven imagery. Arch Gen Psychiatry 53:380–387, 1996

Rauch SL, Whalen PJ, Shin LM, et al: Exaggerated amygdala response to masked facial stimuli in posttraumatic stress disorder: a functional MRI study. Biol Psychiatry 47:769–776, 2000

Rodriguez NR, Ryan SW, Rowan AB, et al: Posttraumatic stress disorder in a clinical sample of adult survivors of childhood sexual abuse. Child Abuse Negl 20:943–952, 1996

Rodriguez NR, Ryan SW, Vande Kemp H, et al: Posttraumatic stress disorder in adult female survivors of child sexual abuse: a comparison study. J Consult Clin Psychol 65:53–59, 1997

Roesler TA, McKenzie N: Effects of childhood trauma on psychological functioning in adults sexually abused as children. J Nerv Ment Dis 182:145–150, 1994

Roth S, Wayland K, Woolsey M: Victimization history and victim-assailant relationship as factors in recovery from sexual assault. J Trauma Stress 3:169–180, 1990

Roth S, Newman E, Pelcovitz D, et al: Complex PTSD in victims exposed to sexual and physical abuse: results from the DSM-IV field trial for posttraumatic stress disorder. J Trauma Stress 10:539–555, 1997

Russell DEH: The Secret Trauma: Incest in the Lives of Girls and Women. New York, Basic Books, 1986

Sack WH, Clark G, Him C, et al: A 6-year follow-up study of Cambodian refugee adolescents traumatized as children. J Am Acad Child Adolesc Psychiatry 32:431–437, 1993

Schaaf KK, McCanne TR: Relationship of childhood sexual, physical, and combined sexual and physical abuse to adult victimization and posttraumatic stress disorder. Child Abuse Negl 22:1119–1133, 1998

Schwartz E, Kowalski J: Posttraumatic stress disorder after a school shooting: effects of symptom threshold selection and diagnosis by DSM-III, DSM-III-R or proposed DSM-IV. Am J Psychiatry 148:592–597, 1991

Sedney MA, Brooks B: Factors associated with a history of childhood sexual experience in a nonclinical female population. Journal of the American Academy of Child Psychiatry 23:215–218, 1984

Selye H: Thymus and adrenals in the response of the organisms to injuries and intoxications. Br J Exp Pathol 17:234–246, 1936

Selye H: The Stress of Life. New York, McGraw-Hill, 1956

Semple WE, Goyer PF, McCormick R, et al: Attention and regional cerebral blood flow in posttraumatic stress disorder patients with substance abuse histories. Psychiatr Res Neuroimaging 67:17–28, 1996

Shannon M, Lonigan C, Finch A, et al: Children exposed to disaster, I: epidemiology of posttraumatic symptoms and symptom profile. J Am Acad Child Adolesc Psychiatry 33:80–93, 1994

Shaw J, Applegate B, Tanner S, et al: Psychological correlates of Hurricane Andrew on an elementary school population. J Am Acad Child Adolesc Psychiatry 34:1185–1192, 1995

Shin LM, McNally RJ, Kosslyn SM, et al: Am J Psychiatry 156:575–584, 1999

Silverman AB, Reinherz HZ, Giaconia RM: The long-term sequelae of child and adolescent abuse: a longitudinal community study. Child Abuse Negl 120: 709–723, 1996

Sorenson SB, Siegel JM, Golding JM, et al: Repeated sexual victimization. Violence and Victims 6:299–308, 1991

Southwick SM, Krystal JH, Morgan CA, et al: Abnormal noradrenergic function in posttraumatic stress disorder. Arch Gen Psychiatry 50:266–274, 1993

Stein JA, Golding JM, Siegel JM, et al: Long-term psychological sequelae of child sexual abuse: the Los Angeles Epidemiologic Catchment Area Study, in Lasting Effects of Child Sexual Abuse. Edited by Wyatt GE, Powell GJ. Newbury Park, CA, Sage Publications, 1988, pp 135–154

Stein MB, Yehuda R, Koverola C, et al: Enhanced dexamethasone suppression of plasma cortisol in adult women traumatized by childhood sexual abuse. Biol Psychiatry 42:680–686, 1997a

Stein MB, Koverola C, Hanna C, et al: Hippocampal volume in women victimized by childhood sexual abuse. Psychol Med 27:951–959, 1997b

Styron T, Janoff-Bulman R: Childhood attachment and abuse: long-term effects on adult attachment, depression, and conflict resolution. Child Abuse Negl 21:1015–1023, 1997

Swett C, Cohen C, Surrey H, et al: High rates of alcohol use and history of physical and sexual abuse among women outpatients. American Journal of Drug and Alcohol Abuse 17:49–60, 1991

Teicher MH, Glod CA, Surrey J, et al: Early childhood abuse and limbic system ratings in adult psychiatric outpatients. J Neuropsychiatry Clin Neurosci 5:301–306, 1993

Teicher MH, Ito Y, Glod CA, et al: Neurophysiological mechanisms of stress response in children, in Severe Stress and Mental Disturbance in Children. Edited by Pfeffer CR. Washington, DC, American Psychiatric Press, 1996, pp 59–84

Terr LC: Psychic trauma in children: observations following the Chowchilla school bus kidnapping. Am J Psychiatry 138:14–19, 1981

Terr LC: Childhood traumas: an outline and overview: Am J Psychiatry 148:10–20, 1991

Thakkar RR, McCanne TR: The effects of daily stressors on physical health in women with and without a childhood history of sexual abuse. Child Abuse Negl 24:209–221, 2000

Triffleman EG, Marmar CR, Delucchi KL, et al: Childhood trauma and posttraumatic stress disorder in substance abuse inpatients. J Nerv Ment Dis 183:172–176, 1995

Tsai M, Feldman-Summers S, Edgar M: Childhood molestation: variables related to differential impacts on psychosexual functioning in adult women. J Abnorm Psychol 88: 407–417, 1979

Tyano S, Iancu I, Solomon Z, et al: Seven-year follow-up of child survivors of a bus–train collision. J Am Acad Child Adolesc Psychiatry 35:365–373, 1996

van der Kolk BA, Perry C, Herman JL: Childhood origins of self-destructive behavior. Am J Psychiatry 148:1665–1671, 1991

Weiss EL, Longhurst JG, Mazure CM: Childhood sexual abuse as a risk factor for depression in women: psychosocial and neurobiological correlates. Am J Psychiatry 156:816–828, 1999

Wenninger K, Ehlers A: Dysfunctional cognitions and adult psychological functioning in child sexual abuse survivors. J Trauma Stress 11:281–300, 1998

Widom CS: Posttraumatic stress disorder in abused and neglected children grown up. Am J Psychiatry 156:1223–1229, 1999

Widom CS, Weiler BL, Cottler LB: Childhood victimization and drug abuse: a comparison of prospective and retrospective findings. J Consult Clin Psychol 67:867–880, 1999

Wind TW, Silvern L: Parenting and family abuse as mediators of the long-term effects of child abuse. Child Abuse Negl 18:439–453, 1994

Winje D, Ulvik A: Long-term outcome of trauma in children: the psychological consequences of a bus accident. J Child Psychol Psychiatry 39:635–642, 1998

Wyatt GE, Newcomb M: Internal and external mediators of women's sexual abuse in childhood. J Consult Clin Psychol 58:758–767, 1990

Yehuda R, Antelman SM: Criteria for rationally evaluating animal models of posttraumatic stress disorder. Biol Psychiatry 33:479–486, 1993

Yehuda R, Southwick SM, Nussbaum G, et al: Low urinary cortisol excretion in patients with posttraumatic stress disorder. J Nerv Ment Dis 178:366–369, 1990

Yehuda R, Southwick SM, Krystal JH, et al: Enhanced suppression of cortisol following dexamethasone administration in posttraumatic stress disorder. Am J Psychiatry 150:83–86, 1993a

Yehuda R, Boisoneau D, Mason JW, et al: Relationship between lymphocyte glucocorticoid receptor number and urinary free cortisol excretion in mood, anxiety, and psychotic disorder. Biol Psychiatry 34:18–25, 1993b

Yehuda R, Boisoneau D, Lowy MT, et al: Dose-response changes in plasma cortisol and lymphocyte glucocorticoid receptors following dexamethasone administration in combat veterans with and without posttraumatic stress disorder. Arch Gen Psychiatry 52:583–593, 1995a

Yehuda R, Kahana B, Schmeidler J, et al: The impact of cumulative lifetime trauma and recent stress on current posttraumatic stress disorder symptoms in Holocaust survivors. Am J Psychiatry 152:1815–1818, 1995b

Yehuda R, Kahana B, Binder-Brynes K, et al: Low urinary cortisol excretion in Holocaust survivors with posttraumatic stress disorder. Am J Psychiatry 152:982–986, 1995c

Yehuda R, Teicher MH, Trestman RL, et al: Cortisol regulation in posttraumatic stress disorder and major depression: a chronobiological analysis. Biol Psychiatry 40:79–88, 1996

Yehuda R, Schmeidler J, Siever LS, et al: Individual differences in posttraumatic stress disorder symptom profiles in Holocaust survivors in concentration camps or in hiding. J Trauma Stress 10:453–463, 1997

Yehuda R, Siever LJ, Teicher MH, et al: Plasma norepinephrine and 3-methoxy-4-hydroxyphenylglycol concentrations and severity of depression in combat posttraumatic stress disorder and major depressive disorder. Biol Psychiatry 44:56–63, 1998

Yehuda R, Bierer LM, Schmeidler J, et al: Low cortisol and risk for PTSD in adult offspring of holocaust survivors. Am J Psychiatry 157:1252–1259, 2000

Zlotnick C: Posttraumatic stress disorder (PTSD), PTSD comorbidity, and childhood abuse among incarcerated women. J Nerv Ment Dis 185:761–763, 1997

Zlotnick C, Zakriski AL, Shea MT, et al: The long-term sequelae of sexual abuse: support for a complex posttraumatic stress disorder. J Trauma Stress 9:195–205, 1996

Index

Page numbers printed in **boldface** type refer to tables

Abuse, sleeper effects of, 128. *See*
    Sexual abuse. *See also* Child
    abuse
Accidents. *See also* Traumatic
    events
    and childhood PTSD, 42
    and PTSD rates, 128
Achenbach Child Behavior
    Checklist (CBCL), 18
Acronym, PTSD, 34
Adjustment disorders, 38
Adolescence, PTSD in, 41
Adolescent Dissociative
    Experiences Scale, 23
Adolescents. *See also* Youth
    at risk, 3
    clinical interview of, 19–21
    nefazodone in, 100
    substance use disorders in, 43
Adrenergic blockers, 74
Adrenocorticotropic hormone
    (ACTH)
    and early stress, 133
    and stress reactivity, 138
Adult facilities, incarceration of
    juveniles in, 77
Adults
    delayed reactions of, 129
    effects of early trauma on, 124

exposed to childhood
    maltreatment, 137
impact of childhood trauma
    on, 117
survivors of child abuse, 131
Affective disorders, in juvenile
    justice population, 61
African-American children,
    PTSD among incarcerated, 67
Age
    and lifetime DSM-IV diagnosis
    of PTSD, 104
    and response to trauma, 40
Aggression, and exposure to
    violence, 66–67
Agitation, in childhood PTSD, 34
Alcohol abuse, 73
    in adolescence, 41
    PTSD associated with, 140
Alprazolam, 101
American Academy of Child and
    Adolescent Psychiatry
    (AACAP)
    assessment standards of, 46
    practice parameters published
    by, 4–5, 16
Amitriptyline, 103
Amnesia
    in Holocaust survivors, 143

Amnesia *(continued)*
  psychogenic, 47
  traumatic, 19
Amygdala
  in fear response, 139
  in threat assessment, 138
Anger, clinical scales for, 15
Animal experiments, on response
  to stress, 134–135
Anticonvulsants, 102
Antipsychotics, 101–102
Anxiety
  clinical scales for, 15
  early trauma associated
    with, 119
  phobic, 126–127
Anxiety disorders, 38, 39
  comorbid with PTSD, 89
  in juvenile justice
    population, 61
Anxiety Disorders Interview
  Schedule, 18
Assessment instruments, 3, 5
  CAPA-PTSD, 5–7
  CAPS-CA, 7–9, 96, 104
  CPTSDI, 9–10
  CPTS-RI, 10–12
  Darryl, 12–14
  in forensic examination, 45–46
  K-SADS-PL, 12, 18
  in Spanish, 18
  TSCC, 14–15
Assessment, PTSD, 2
  clinical, 4, 5–15
  clinical interview in, 16–21
  cognitive assessment, 21–22,
    26
  developmental issues in, 2–3
  and diagnostic criteria, 1–2, 3
  emotional functioning in, 22
  forensic examination in, 45–47

  multidimensional approach to,
    15–25
  overreliance on DSM-IV
    criteria, 4
  projective techniques, 24–25, 26
  self-report measures, 23–24
Attention deficit disorders, in
  juvenile justice population,
  61
Attention-deficit/hyperactivity
  disorder (ADHD), 99
  diagnosis of, 36, 37
  risperidone for, 102
Augmentation strategies, in
  PTSD, 102
Autonomic nervous system, 133
Avoidance symptoms
  age and, 40
  manifestation of, 71
  in PTSD diagnosis, 34, 35

Behavioral observations, in PTSD
  assessment, 16–17
Benzodiazepines, 51, 92
  in children, 74
  contraindication for, 90
Bereavement, treatment for, 71
β-blockers, for PTSD symptoms,
  98–99. *See also* Propranolol
Biological treatment
  α2-agonists, 98
  anticonvulsants, 99–100
  beta blockers, 98
  for childhood PTSD, 94–95
  with MAOIs, 97–98
  with SSRIs, 95
  with TCAs, 97–98
Bipolar disorders
  in juvenile justice population, 61
  risperidone for, 102
Brain, dysfunction of, 48

Brain regions, implicated in
    PTSD, 90–91
Brain size, in maltreated children,
    140
Brain volume, and PTSD, 91
Buffalo Creek disaster, 34,
    125–126
Buspirone, 100, 102

California Youth Authority
    (CYA), 63
Cancer, childhood, and PTSD
    incidence, 42, 43
Capacity, determination of
    mental, 52
Carbamazepine, 94, 99, 100
Case management, 73
Catecholamines
    in adults with PTSD, 136
    in maltreated children with
        PTSD, 137
Census of Juveniles in
    Residential Placement
    (CJRP), 60
Center for Mental Health
    Services, of DHHS, 59
Cerebellum, in threat assessment,
    138. *See also* Brain
Child abuse
    adult survivors of, 131
    recovered adult memories of, 48
Child and Adolescent Psychiatric
    Assessment: Life Events
    Section and PTSD Module
    (CAPA-PTSD), 5–7
Child Depression Inventory
    (CDI), 23
Child Dissociative Checklist
    (CDC), 23
Childhood Trauma
    Questionnaire, 23

Child Interview Schedule, 18
Child Posttraumatic Stress
    Reaction Index (CPTS-RI)
    description, 10–11
    psychometric properties of, 11
Child PTSD Symptom Scale
    (CPSS), 104
Children
    clinical interviews of, 19–21
    PTSD in incarcerated, 63
Children, maltreated, brain size
    and, 140. *See also*
    Maltreatment, childhood
Children's Apperception Test
    (CAT), 25
Children's Depression Rating
    Scale–Revised (CDRS-R), 20
Children's PTSD Inventory
    (CPTSDI)
    description, 9–10
    validation study for, 10
Children's Self-Report and
    Projective Inventory (CSRPI),
    25
Children, traumatized,
    longitudinal examinations of,
    127. *See also* Trauma,
    childhood
Chloral hydrate treatment, 98
Chowchilla kidnapping incident,
    34
Chronicity, of PTSD syndromes, 50
Cingulum
    in threat assessment, 138
    in trauma-exposed subjects, 139
Circadian rhythmicity, enhanced,
    138
Citalopram treatment, 96–97
Clinical Global Impression (CGI)
    Scale, 95, 96, 102
Clinical trials, 90

Clinician-Administered PTSD
Scale for Children and
Adolescents (CAPS-CA),
7–9, 96, 104
description, 7–8
psychometric properties of, 9
reliability and validity for, 9
Clonazepam, 74, 101
Clonidine, 51, 74, 93, 94, 99, 102
Clonidine patches, 99
Cognitive assessment, 21–22, 26
Cognitive-behavioral
psychotherapy, 50
Cognitive-behavioral treatment
(CBT), 94–95
efficacy of, 106
in imipramine study, 98
Cognitive function, and PTSD, 43
Combat veterans. *See also*
Vietnam War veterans
studies with, 103, 104
yohimbine probe in, 92
Communities, PTSD intervention
in, 76
Community programming, and
recidivism rates, 72
Comorbidity
with PTSD, 3, 68
rates of, 39
Compounded community
trauma, 66
Conduct disorders
among juvenile justice
populations, 61
risperidone for, 102
Corticosterone secretion, and
early stress, 133
Corticotropin releasing factor
(CRF)
in animal experiments, 134
in PTSD, 91

Cortisol levels, 91–92
in maltreated children with
PTSD, 137
in PTSD, 136
Criminal justice system, and
mental health issues, 60
Criminal records, reports of
abuse in, 130
Cultural factors, and PTSD
manifestation, 43–44, 67, 68
Custodial staff, traumatized, 73
Cyproheptadine, 100

Darryl instrument
design, 12–13
future field testing for, 13–14
reliability and validity of,
13
Defensive behavior, in evaluation
process, 2
Delinquency offenses, youth
charged with, 60
Demographics, of juvenile justice
systems, 60, 65, 78
Depression
clinical scales for, 15
early trauma associated
with, 119
and exposure to single
traumatic event, 126–127
Depressive disorders, 39
PTSD associated with, 43
risperidone for, 102
Desensitization phenomena, 72
Desensitization techniques, 73
Desipramine, 97
Detachment, in Holocaust
survivors, 143
Detention facilities
intervention for PTSD in, 75
women and girls in, 77

Developmental disorders,
    in juvenile justice population,
    61
Dexamethasone, cortisol
    response to, 133, 134
Diagnosis, PTSD, 34–38
    age and, 104
    criterion A for, 34, 38
    criterion B for, 35
    criterion C for, 35–36
    criterion D for, 36
    differential diagnoses for, 36
    and phenomenology, 88–90
*Diagnostic and Statistical Manual of
    Mental Disorders* (DSM),
    33–34. *See also* DSM-II,
    DSM-III, DSM-III-R, DSM-IV
Diagnostic Interview for
    Children and Adolescents–
    Revised, 20–21
Diagnostic Interview Schedule
    for Children–Supplemental
    PTSD Module, 21
Disasters
    Buffalo Creek, 34, 124–126
    exposure to community, 62
    exposure to natural, 62
    and PTSD rates, 128
Disorganized behavior, in
    childhood PTSD, 34
Dissociation
    early trauma associated
        with, 119
    in Holocaust survivors, 143
Dissociative symptoms
    clinical scales for, 15
    treatment of, 72
Distress, and PTSD criteria,
    67–68
Domestic violence, and PTSD
    rates, 128

Dopamine, and PTSD
    symptoms, 93
Dopamine blocking agents,
    101–102
Dopaminergic system, in PTSD, 93
Draw-A-Person projective
    technique, 20
Drawing activities
    for adolescents, 73
    in evaluation with young
        children, 19–20
Dreams, adults' vs. children's, 2
Drug abuse, in adolescence, 41.
    See also Substance abuse
Drug therapy, efficacy of, 106. *See
    also* Pharmacotherapy
DSM-II, 34
DSM-III, 1, 7, 34
DSM-III-R, 7
DSM-IV
    CAPS-CA for, 7–9
    diagnosis of PTSD in, 34, 44
    PTSD in, 88, 142
Dysfunctional family, and PTSD
    symptoms, 68
Dysfunctional interpersonal
    relationships, in assessment
    outcomes, 105

Earthquake, Armenian, response
    of adolescents to, 136
Efficacy, of drug therapy, 90, 103,
    106
Emotional detachment, in
    Holocaust survivors, 143
Emotional functioning,
    assessment of, 23
Epidemiologic Catchment Area
    study, 38, 62
Epidemiology, PTSD, 38–39
Ethnic cleansing, exposure to, 142

Ethnicity, and disparity in confinement of juvenile offenders, 77–78

Evaluation, PTSD. *See also* Assessment

bias in, 46

cognitive assessment in, 21–22, 26

forensic, 51

multi-dimensional approach in, 15

prospective vs. retrospective, 144

time factors in, 2

Exposure to early trauma, and adult PTSD symptoms, 118. *See also* Traumatic events

Eye movement desensitization, 50

Eye movement desensitization and reprocessing (EMDR), 73

Families

in PTSD interventions, 75

significant problems with, 131

supportive relationships of, 68

Family planning, 77

Fluoxetine, 95, 102

in adults, 103

for PTSD symptoms, 96

Fluvoxamine trials, 96

Forensic examination, in PTSD assessment, 45–47

Forensic expert, role of, 46

Forensic issues, 4

Forensic psychiatrist, 33

Foster care, and child trauma cases, 41–42

Four studies, the, 63, **64**

female subjects in, 65

racial/ethnic distribution in, 68

substance use in, 67

Freudian paradigm, for adult trauma victims, 33

GABA pathways, in PTSD, 93–94

Gabapentin, 99

Gang membership, of incarcerated youth, 69

Gender differences

in exposure to trauma, 88

in juvenile offenses, 60

in psychological symptoms related to early trauma, **120–123**

in PTSD occurrence, 39–40

Genetics

effect of stressors on, 132, 133

of PTSD, 39

Girls, in juvenile justice system, 65. *See also* Women

Glucocorticoid receptor concentrations, and early stress, 133–134

Glutamergic pathways

biologic dysregulation of, 87

in PTSD, 93–94

Grief, treatment for, 71

Gross stress reaction, 34

Group treatment techniques, in juvenile justice population, 73

Guanfacine, 94, 99

Guilt, in assessment outcomes, 105

Gun involvement, of incarcerated youth, 69

Gunshot wounds, 66

Health and Human Services (HHS), U.S. Dept. of, Center for Mental Health Services of, 59

Hippocampus
    examination of volume, 139–140
    in threat assessment, 138

Holocaust, survivors of European
    hypervigilance in, 143
    PTSD in, 141

Home life, negative, and prostitution, 41. *See also* Families

Homicide, witnessing
    and PTSD development, 69
    and PTSD rates, 128

House-Tree-Person test, 19–20

Hyperarousal symptoms
    age and, 40
    misdiagnosis of, 37
    in PTSD diagnosis, 34

Hypervigilance, in Holocaust survivors, 143

Hypothalamic-pituitary-adrenal (HPA) axis, 133
    alterations of, 91
    impact of early adverse events on, 135
    in PTSD, 137
    in response to traumatic events, 136
    and stress reactivity, 138

Illness, early trauma associated with, 124

Imaging studies
    of brain function and behavior, 138–139
    MRI, 91
    techniques, 50

Imipramine, 95, 98

Immigrants, and PTSD, 43–44

Impact of Events Scale (IES), 23

Index
    Child Posttraumatic Stress Reaction, 10–12
    PTSD Reaction (self-report), 104

Information, stored in memory, 49

Integrated service delivery approach, for juveniles, 79

Integration of affect, 24

Intercourse, forced, 65

Interpersonal problems
    assessment of, 105
    early trauma associated with, 124

Interventions for PTSD
    community, 76–77
    family, 75
    group, 73
    individual, 70
    pharmacotherapy, 73–74

Interview protocol, for physical abuse data, 71

Interviews
    face-to-face, 15, 26
    semistructured, 20–21

Interview Schedule for Children and Adolescents, 21

Interviews, clinical, 16–17
    of children and adolescents, 19–21
    of parents, 17–19
    structured, 21, 45–46

Inventories
    children's PTSD, 9
    Children's Self-Report and Projective (CSRPI), 25
    Minnesota Multiphasic Personality (MMPI), 4, 18–19, 46
    YSR, 18

Israel, long-term impact of
     terrorist attack in, 126

Justice, U.S. Dept. of, Civil Rights
     Division of, 59
Juvenile Justice and Delinquency
     Prevention Act (1974), 78
Juvenile justice facilities, national
     survey of, 59
Juvenile justice system, 59
     clinical assessments in, 70
     demographics for, 60, 65
     prevalence of mental disorders
          in, 61–62
     women and girls in, 65
Juveniles, defined, 60

Kiddie MMPI, 18
Kiddie Schedule for Affective
     Disorders and Schizophrenia
     for School-Age Children–
     Present and Lifetime Version
     (K-SADS-PL), 12, 18
Kiddie Schedule for Affective
     Disorders and Schizophrenia
     for School-age Children
     (K-SADS), 18
Kidnapping
     Chowchilla incident, 34
     and PTSD rates, 128

Lamotrigine, 99
Latino children, and PTSD, 43–44
Learning disabilities, in juvenile
     justice population, 61
Life Events Checklist (LEC), 8
Life Events Section (LES), of
     CAPA, 6
Limbic system dysfunction, and
     early abuse, 140
Lithium carbonate, 102

Lymphocyte glucocorticoid
     receptors, in PTSD, 91, 137

Magnetic resonance imaging
     study, PTSD in, 91
Maltreatment, childhood
     brain size and, 140
     diverse effects of, 146
     exposure to, 62
     long-term consequences of,
          118–124
     and maternal history of
          abuse, 145
     and MRI study, 91
     neuroanatomic studies in
          adults exposed to, 138–141
     and neuroendocrine
          findings, 136
     and psychologic symptoms,
          120–123
     stress reactivity in adults
          exposed to, 137–138
     survivors of, 137
     and victimization, 129–131
Marijuana abuse, 73
Massachusetts Youth Screening
     Instrument–2nd Revision, 70
Maternal deprivation
     and coping with adversity,
          134–135
     physiological responses
          associated with, 134
M-chlorophenylpiperazine
     (m-CPP), 93
Medical-legal expert, 46
Medications, 103. *See also*
     Biological treatment;
     Pharmacotherapy
     benzodiazepines, 101
     dopamine blocking agents for,
          101–102

efficacy of, 106
lithium carbonate, 102
opioid antagonists, 101
psychotherapy facilitated
by, 95
for PTSD, 94–95
serotonergic agents, 100–101
stimulant, 37
Memory
components of, 49
disturbances of, 48
forensic aspects of, 54
inaccurate postevent data in, 49
PTSD and, 47–50
recovered, 33, 50
for traumatic events, 143–144
Mental disorders
and justice system, 76
prevalence of, 61
Mental Health Juvenile Justice
Act, 60
Mental health symptoms
after single-event traumatic
episode, 126
in criminal justice system, 60
Mental illness, and veracity of
report, 50
Methodology, in study of long-
term impact of childhood
trauma, 143–146
Methylphenidate, 102
Metyrapone administration, 91
MHPG (3-methoxy-
4-hydroxyphenylglycol),
in PTSD, 136
Minnesota Multiphasic
Personality Inventory
(MMPI), 19
Minnesota Multiphasic
Personality Inventory-2
(MMPI-2), 46

Minnesota Multiphasic
Personality Inventory–
Adolescent (MMPI-A), 4, 24
Minority populations. *See also*
Women
African-American children, 67
in juvenile justice system, 78
Latino children, 43–44
Mistrust, in assessment
outcomes, 105
Moclobemide, 98
Molecular biology, 104
Molecular neurobiologic
studies, 132
Monoamine oxidase inhibitors
(MAOIs), 51
for PTSD symptoms, 97–98
and reexperience phenomena,
74
Mood disorders
among incarcerated youth, 79
PTSD comorbid with, 89
Mothers. *See also* Women
abused women as, 145
of children with cancer, 42
effect on childhood PTSD of, 54
and resilience of children, 44
Motor cortex, in threat
assessment, 138
Motor vehicle accidents, and
childhood PTSD, 42
Multi-Systemic Therapy Model, 76
Murderers, juvenile, 61
Murder, witnessing, 128

Naloxone, 101
National Comorbidity Study, 38
National Women's Study, 40
Near-miss phenomenon, 66
Needle sticks, as stressors, 132
Nefazodone, 100, 103

Negative feedback inhibition, exaggerated, 138
Neuroanatomy, in adults exposed to childhood maltreatment, 138–141
Neurobiologic systems, 90–94
neuroendocrine alterations in, 91–92
neurotransmission, 92–94
Neurocognitive impairment, in juvenile justice population, 61. *See also* Cognitive assessment
Neuroendocrine system
alterations in PTSD, 91–92
pathways of, 87
responses to stress of, 134
Neurophysiology, forensic aspects of, 54
Neuropsychologist
on PTSD assessment team, 16
in PTSD evaluations, 21–22
Neurotransmitter systems
dopamine, 93
GABA, 93–94
glutamate, 93–94
norepinephrine, 92–93
serotonin, 93
Night terrors, 26
Nightmares
abuse and, 145
relieving, 100
Noradrenergic agents, 97
Noradrenergic systems
impact of early adverse events on, 135
pathways for, 87
in PTSD, 92
Norepinephrine, in neurotransmission, 92–93
Numbing, in PTSD diagnosis, 34, 35. *See also* Symptoms

Olanzapine, 101
Opiates, 92
Opioid antagonists, 101
Oppositional defiant disorders, risperidone for, 102
Outcome, assessing, 104–105
Overreporting, of emotional trauma, 47

Panic attacks, m-CPP-induced, 93
Panic disorders
clonazepam for, 74
TCAs in, 98
Parenting instruction, 77
Parents
and affect modulation, 43
clinical interview with, 17, 26
in juvenile justice system, 77
symptomatology of, 69
Parietal cortex, in threat assessment, 138
Paroxetine, 96
Path analysis, 131
Persian Gulf War, 127
Personality
assessment of, 23
and repeated exposure to trauma, 71
and trauma-related expectations, 47
Personality disorders, early trauma associated with, 119
Personality inventories, 4, 19, 24, 46
Personality Inventory for Children (PIC), 4, 18
Pharmacogenetics, 104
Pharmacotherapy, 50, 51. *See also* Medications
effectiveness of, 90, 103
predictors of response to, 103–104

for PTSD, 73–74
symptom clusters as target for, 89
Phenelzine, 98
Phobic anxiety, and exposure to single traumatic event, 126–127
Physical abuse
and PTSD development, 117
vs. single-episode events, 125
Physical abuse, childhood
lack of support in, 129
and PTSD in adults, 128
Physical anomalies, violent delinquency associated with, 67–68
Physical illness, early trauma associated with, 124
Physiology
effects of stress on, 132
of PTSD, 44–45
Play therapy, 73
Political oppression, exposure to, 142
Posttraumatic stress disorder (PTSD)
among incarcerated youth, 63, **64,** 65
appropriate treatment for, 103
clinical assessment of, 5
cognitive processing in, 141
comorbidity with, 3
in DSM-IV, 34, 88
diagnosis of, 33
interventions for, 70–77
introduction of, 34
lifetime diagnosis of, 62
neurobiologic systems in, 90–94
partial, 63
predisposing factors for, 65–69
prevalence of, 39–39, 127–129
psychobiologic dysfunction in, 87–88
and quality of life, 105
risk factors for, 131
variation in rates of, 127–128
Posttraumatic stress disorder (PTSD), childhood
age-specific symptoms in, 3
diagnosis of, 34–38
epidemiology of, 38–39
heritable component to transmission of, 39
and memory, 47–50
other psychiatric disorders associated with, 89
pharmacologic studies of, 105–106
precipitating events in, 3
and psychophysiologic alterations, 44–45
rates of, 62–63
risk factors for, 39–44
severity of, 37
survivors of, 117
treatment of, 50–51
types of, 36
Posttraumatic stress (PTS), clinical scales for, 15
Prevalence, of PTSD, 38–39, 127–129
Projective measures, in PTSD assessment, 24–25, 26
Propranolol, 74, 94
with imipramine, 102
for PTSD symptoms, 98–99
Prostitution, childhood sexual abuse and, 41
Proton magnetic resonance spectroscopy, 139
Psychobiology, of PTSD, 87–88, 94

Psychologic symptoms
 childhood maltreatment and,
  120–123
 methodologic issues in study
  of, 144–145
Psychopathology, trauma-related
 in childhood, 131
 risk factors for, 66
Psychopharmacology, forensic
 aspects of, 54. *See also*
 Biological treatment
Psychophysiology, of PTSD, 44–45
Psychosocial interventions, 50
Psychotherapy
 with biological treatment, 95
 cognitive-behavioral, 50
Psychotic disturbances
 in juvenile justice population, 61
 risperidone for, 102
Psychoticism, and single-episode
 traumatic event, 127
Psychotropic agents, 74
PTSD module, of CAPA, 6–7
PTSD Reaction Index
 (self-report), 104
PTSD Scale, Clinician-
 Administered, 7–9
PTSD syndrome, 40

Quality of life, 105
Quetiapine, 101

Race, and disparity in
 confinement of juvenile
 offenders, 77–78
Rape victims, and childhood
 sexual assault, 130. *See also*
 Women, abused
Reality testing, 24
Recidivism, community
 programming and, 72

Recovery, variation in rates of, 128
Reenactment behaviors, in
 childhood PTSD, 35
Reexperiencing symptoms
 age and, 40
 in PTSD diagnosis, 34
Rehabilitation, community-
 based, 76
Relaxation techniques, 73
Remedial education, 77
Resistant behaviors, in
 evaluation process, 2
Retraumatization, 20, 117, 146.
 See also Revictimization
Retrospective studies, of early
 maltreatment, 146
Revenge fantasies, 71
Revictimization, impact of early
 maltreatment on, 129–131
Revised Children's Manifest
 Anxiety Scale (RCMAS), 23
Reynolds Adolescent Depression
 Scale, 23
Risk factors for PTSD, 39
 need to delineate, 146
 and symptoms, 68
Risperidone, 101, 102
Roberts Apperception Test for
 Children (RATC), 25
Roleplay, in clinical interview, 19
Rorschach Inkblot Test, 24
Rotter Incomplete Sentence
 Blank, 25

School, intervention for PTSD
 in, 75
SCUD missiles, 127
Seizures, kindled, 132
Selective serotonin reuptake
 inhibitors (SSRIs), 103
 for adult PTSD, 51, 95

safety profiles of, 97
Self-report checklists, 46
Self-report measures, 23–24
Sensitization, time-dependent, 132
Sentence Completion Series
(SCS), 25
Serotonergic agents, 94, 100–101
Serotonergic pathways, 87, 93
Sertraline, 95–96
Sexual abuse
emotional sequelae of, 52
neurophysiologic markers
of, 45
and PTSD development, 117
vs. single-episode events, 125
Sexual abuse, childhood
and adult reaction to stress,
137–138
adult survivors of, 47–48
and adult vulnerability, 131
lack of support in, 129
pathologic memories of, 48
psychological sequelae of, 145
and PTSD in adults, 128
trauma associated with, 41
Sexual assault victims,
revictimization of, 130
Sexual concerns, clinical scales
for, 15
Sexual dysfunction
early childhood sexual abuse
associated with, 128
and early trauma, 119, 124
Sexual precocity, and
prostitution, 41
Shame, in assessment outcomes,
105
Shooting, exposure to, 66. *See also*
Gun involvement
Sleeper effects, of abuse, 128
Sodium valproate, 99

Somatoform disorders, and
exposure to single traumatic
event, 126–127
Spanish
assessment instruments in, 18
self-report measures in, 23
Stabbing, exposure to, 66
Standardization and reliability
data, for PTSD module, 7
Statistical probability mapping,
of brain function and
behavior, 138–139
Status offenses, youth charged
with, 60. *See also* Youth,
incarcerated
Stimulant medications, 37
Stress. *See* Traumatic stress. *See
also* Traumatic events
biological models of effects of,
132–133
developmental influences of
early, 133
and gene products, 132
intergenerational effects of, 133
lifelong implications of, 132–133
multilayered, 35
Stress management techniques,
72, 75
Stress theory, 132
Subjective data, reliance on,
143–144
Substance abuse
among incarcerated youth, 67
among juvenile justice
population, 79
early trauma associated
with, 119
intergenerational pattern of, 67
PTSD associated with, 140
and single-episode traumatic
events, 126

Substance use disorders, comorbid
   with PTSD, 39, 43, 89
Suggestibility, and retrieval of
   information, 49
Suicidal ideation
   among incarcerated youth, 69
   early trauma associated
      with, 119
   monitoring of, 71
   and single-episode traumatic
      events, 126
Survivor guilt, 7
Survivors, Holocaust, 141–143,
   141–143
Survivors, trauma
   hippocampal volume in,
      139–140
   hyperresponsivity to stress
      of, 134
   neuroanatomic studies in, 138
Symptom Checklist-90, 143
Symptoms, PTSD, 2
   α2-agonists for, 99
   acute vs. chronic, 89
   among mental health
      problems, 118
   anticonvulsants for, 99–100
   β-blockers for, 98
   decline over time, 127, 128
   dopamine blocking agents for,
      101–102
   gender differences in, 39–40
   MAOIs for, 97–98
   opioid antagonists for, 101
   serotonergic agents for, 100–101
   and single-episode traumatic,
      127
   SSRIs for, 95–97
   TCAs for, 97
   triad of, 38
Syndrome, PTSD, 40

Tardive dyskinesia, 102
Team, PTSD assessment, 16
Terrorist attack, long-term impact
   of, 126
Testimony, child victim, 33
   distortion of, 50
   forensic aspects of, 54
   in sexual abuse cases, 48
Testimony, expert, 51
Test results, limitations of, 26
Thematic Apperception Test
   (TAT), 25
Thioridazine, 101
Transient situational disturbance,
   34
Trauma
   and child's development, 66
   enduring effects of, 124
   exposure rates, 87
   PTSD-precipitating, 8
   type II reactions, 66
   types causing childhood
      PTSD, 38
Trauma, childhood
   biological consequences in
      adults of, 135–141
   classification of, 89
   longitudinal examinations of,
      127
   long-term impact of, 143–146
   and memory, 48
Trauma, response to, 40
   impact of early maltreatment
      on, 129–131
   psychophysiologic alterations
      in, 44
Trauma Symptom Checklist
   for Children (TSCC), 4,
      14–15, 23
Traumatic events
   exploration of, 71–72

functional impairment
associated with, 78
long-term consequences of,
125–127
memory for, 143–144
neurohormonal release in, 141
recollections of, 145
single vs. chronic, 142
single-episode, 125
Traumatic stress
duration of, 35
and personality, 47
Trazodone, 100
Treatment, for PTSD, 51
Tricyclic antidepressants
(TCAs), 94
efficacy of, 74
for PTSD symptoms, 97–98

Underreporting
of child's distress, 17
of emotional trauma, 47

Validity scales
in cognitive assessment, 26
for PIC, 19
for TSCC, 23
Veterans Affairs, U.S. Dept. of,
34
Victimization. *See also*
Revictimization
and mental health evaluations,
79
methodologic issues in study
of, 144
predictors of, 130
and PTSD criteria, 67–68
Vietnam Era Twin Registry, 39
Vietnam War, 33
Vietnam War veterans, brain
studies in, 139

Vineland Adaptive Behavior
Scales–Interview Edition, 17
Violence
community, 66
in home, 75
interpersonal, 142
and PTSD criteria, 67–68
and PTSD symptoms, 68
reactive, 72

War
exposure to, 62, 142
Persian Gulf, 127
and PTSD rates, 128
Wechsler Intelligence Scale for
Children–Third Edition, 22
Women, abused, 137
as mothers, 145
neuroanatomy of, 139–140
stress reactivity of, 137
Women, in juvenile justice system,
65. *See also* Gender differences
World War I, 34

Yohimbine, as noradrenergic
probe, 92
Youth. *See also* juveniles
Youth, incarcerated
in adult facilities, 77
community interventions for,
76–77
family interventions for, 75
group interventions for, 73
individual interventions for,
70–73
Latina females among, 69
pharmacotherapy for, 73–74
PTSD in, 63, **64,** 65
substance abuse among, 67
Youth Self Report inventory
(YSR), 18